Advanced ENT Training

Advanced ENT Training
A Guide to Passing the FRCS
(ORL-HNS) Examination

Edited by

Joseph Manjaly
MBChB BSc (Hons) DOHNS FRCS (ORL-HNS)
Consultant ENT Surgeon
The Royal National ENT Hospital and University
College London Hospitals, United Kingdom

Peter Kullar
MA MB BChir DOHNS MRCS PhD
NIHR Clinical Lecturer and Academic ENT Trainee
Cambridge University Hospitals, United Kingdom

with exam pearls from ENT senior trainees and
consultants from around the United Kingdom

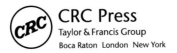

CRC Press
Taylor & Francis Group
Boca Raton London New York

CRC Press is an imprint of the
Taylor & Francis Group, an **informa** business

CRC Press
Taylor & Francis Group
6000 Broken Sound Parkway NW, Suite 300
Boca Raton, FL 33487-2742

© 2020 by Taylor & Francis Group, LLC
CRC Press is an imprint of Taylor & Francis Group, an Informa business

No claim to original U.S. Government works

Printed on acid-free paper

International Standard Book Number-13: 978-0-367-20251-4 (Paperback)

**Visit the Taylor & Francis Web site at
http://www.taylorandfrancis.com**

**and the CRC Press Web site at
http://www.crcpress.com**

For Sarah and Joshua Manjaly

For Kirsty, Max and Cassia Kullar

Contents

Foreword   *xiii*
Editors   *xv*
Senior Section Editors   *xvii*
Contributors   *xix*
Abbreviations   *xxi*

CHAPTER 1 INTRODUCTION   **1**
JOSEPH MANJALY AND PETER KULLAR

**CHAPTER 2 PERSONAL REFLECTIONS ON THE FRCS
(ORL-HNS) PART 1 EXPERIENCE**   **3**
ALISON CARTER

CHAPTER 3 GENERAL ADVICE FOR PREPARING FOR PART 2   **7**
JOSEPH MANJALY

**CHAPTER 4 HISTORIES AND EXAMINATIONS IN THE PART 2
CLINICAL SECTION**   **11**
JOSEPH MANJALY AND PETER KULLAR

Examining the 'Dizzy' Patient   **16**
MANOHAR BANCE

CHAPTER 5 COMMON HEAD AND NECK VIVA TOPICS   **25**
EDITED BY JAMES O'HARA

Benign Laryngeal Lesions   **26**
CHADWAN AL-YAGHCHI

Deep Neck Space Infections   **29**
MOHIEMEN ANWAR

Hypercalcaemia and Hypocalcaemia   **33**
ZI-WEI LIU

Hypopharyngeal Cancer   **35**
LAURA WARNER

Laryngeal Cancer   **38**
LAURA WARNER

Nasopharyngeal Cancer   **42**
JASON FLEMING

Neck Dissection and Accessory Nerve Palsy   **45**
JAGDEEP VIRK

Obstructive Sleep Apnoea (OSA)   **48**
ZI-WEI LIU

Oral Cavity Cancer   **50**
JASON FLEMING

Oropharyngeal Cancer   54
LAURA WARNER

Penetrating Neck Trauma   58
JASON FLEMING

Pharyngeal Pouch   61
JAGDEEP VIRK

Post-laryngectomy Care   64
JASON FLEMING

Post-laryngectomy Complications   67
ZI-WEI LIU

Radiotherapy, Chemotherapy and Osteoradionecrosis   69
JAGDEEP VIRK

Ranula   72
CHADWAN AL-YAGHCHI

Salivary Gland Malignancy   74
JAGDEEP VIRK

Sialolithiasis   77
CHADWAN AL-YAGHCHI

Thyroid Pathology   79
ZI-WEI LIU

Unknown Primary Cancer in the Head and Neck   82
LAURA WARNER

Vocal Cord Palsy   86
CHADWAN AL-YAGHCHI

CHAPTER 6 COMMON OTOLOGY VIVA TOPICS   91
EDITED BY JAMES R TYSOME AND NEIL DONNELLY

Air Conduction Hearing Devices   92
JAMEEL MUZAFFAR AND SUSAN EITUTIS

Benign Paroxysmal Positional Vertigo   94
NICHOLAS DAWE

Bone Conduction Hearing Implants and Middle Ear Implants   98
JAMEEL MUZAFFAR AND JOSEPH MANJALY

Cerebellopontine Angle Tumours   102
NISHCHAY MEHTA

Cholesteatoma   105
NICHOLAS DAWE

Chronic Otitis Media   110
JOSEPH MANJALY

Cochlear Implantation   113
ROBERT NASH AND JOSEPH MANJALY

Ear drops and Anaesthetics 116
JOSEPH MANJALY

Facial Palsy 117
NISHCHAY MEHTA

Ménière's disease 121
KIRAN JUMANI AND PETER KULLAR

Necrotising Otitis Externa 126
NISHCHAY MEHTA

Noise-induced Hearing Loss 129
JAMEEL MUZAFFAR

Non-organic Hearing Loss 132
KIRAN JUMANI

Ossiculoplasty 135
NIKUL AMIN

Otosclerosis 139
JOSEPH MANJALY

Paraganglioma 143
PETER KULLAR

Pre-auricular Sinus 147
NIKUL AMIN

Sensorineural Hearing Loss, Presbyacusis, Autoimmune Hearing Loss 149
NIKUL AMIN

Sudden Sensorineural Hearing Loss 152
NICHOLAS DAWE

Temporal Bone Fracture 156
KIRAN JUMANI AND PETER KULLAR

Tinnitus 160
NISHCHAY MEHTA

Vertigo 162
NICHOLAS DAWE

CHAPTER 7 COMMON PAEDIATRIC ENT VIVA TOPICS 169
EDITED BY BENJAMIN HARTLEY AND RICHARD J HEWITT

Branchial Anomalies 170
JESSICA BEWICK

Cervical Lymphadenopathy 172
JESSICA BEWICK

Choanal Atresia 174
MATTHEW ELLIS

Cleft Lip and Palate 178
SUNIL SHARMA

Congenital Midline Nasal Masses — 182
SUNIL SHARMA

Developmental Milestones, Hearing and Speech, Autism — 184
JESSICA BEWICK

Drooling — 186
GARETH LLOYD

Juvenile Nasopharyngeal Angiofibroma — 188
COLIN BUTLER

Laryngomalacia — 192
MATTHEW ELLIS

Microtia — 195
SUNIL SHARMA

Obstructive Sleep Apnoea — 197
LAKHBINDER PABLA

Otitis Media — 201
ROBERT NASH

Paediatric Airway Compromise — 204
LAKHBINDER PABLA

Paediatric Hearing Loss — 211
ROBERT NASH AND JOSEPH MANJALY

Periorbital Cellulitis — 216
GARETH LLOYD

Recurrent Respiratory Papillomatosis — 220
LAKHBINDER PABLA

Syndromes in ENT — 222
SUNIL SHARMA

Thyroglossal Duct Cyst — 227
JESSICA BEWICK

Tonsillitis and Post-Tonsillectomy Bleeding — 230
GARETH LLOYD

Vascular Malformations — 234
MATTHEW ELLIS

CHAPTER 8 COMMON RHINOLOGY AND FACIAL PLASTICS VIVA TOPICS — 239
EDITED BY HESHAM SALEH

Acute Sinonasal Infections — 240
MOHIEMEN ANWAR

Allergic Rhinitis and Nasal Steroids — 244
THOMAS JACQUES

Anosmia — 248
MARK FERGUSON

Chronic Rhinosinusitis 250
MARK FERGUSON

CSF Rhinorrhoea 253
MOHIEMEN ANWAR

Endoscopic Sinus Surgery 256
MOHIEMEN ANWAR

Epistaxis 259
SAMIT UNADKAT

Facial Flaps and Reconstruction 262
THOMAS JACQUES

Facial Pain 267
THOMAS JACQUES

Fungal Sinusitis 270
MOHIEMEN ANWAR

Hereditary Haemorrhagic Telangiectasia 273
MARK FERGUSON

Keloids 276
THOMAS JACQUES

Olfactory Neuroblastoma 279
MARK FERGUSON

Pinnaplasty 282
SAMIT UNADKAT

Septal Perforation 285
MARK FERGUSON

Septorhinoplasty 288
SAMIT UNADKAT

Sinonasal Tumours 292
MOHIEMEN ANWAR

Skin Cancer 295
SAMIT UNADKAT

Index *299*

Foreword

Joseph Manjaly and Peter Kullar bring energy and enthusiasm to all their endeavours. I know both well following their time in Cambridge. Joseph completed his otology and hearing implant training at Addenbrooke's before taking up a consultant post at the Royal National Throat, Nose and Ear Hospital. Peter is following an academic career and is destined to shape academic otolaryngology over the years to come. Both have a passion and commitment that they want to bring to the task of educating young surgeons, understanding that the FRCS (ORL-HNS) (Fellowship of the Royal Colleges of Surgeons [Otorhinolaryngology – Head and Neck Surgery]) examination is a hurdle that weighs heavily on senior trainees who have so little free time.

Our surgical training programme is not only for learning a curriculum and surgical technique, but also for developing higher order thinking skills that make us problem solvers, deep thinkers, bold innovators, collaborative team players and assertive leaders. It seeks an intrinsic motivation for learning and research to discover the joy in our speciality. My role in ENT training comes towards the senior years – to take a senior trainee and help him or her become an otologist or skull base surgeon equipped to take our speciality forward. But to ensure transformative learning in the final fellowship years there needs to be core knowledge and experience applying that knowledge. The earlier a trainee starts down this road, the more valuable each patient contact becomes.

Advanced ENT Training: A Guide to Passing the FRCS (ORL-HNS) Examination presents insight into an examination that is shrouded in mystery and conflated by half-truths. Joseph and Peter have carefully considered our curriculum and analysed every step of the examination to create a structure for learning that focusses on the task of attaining a good pass. Examiners want concise and well-structured answers about the investigation, diagnosis and management of ENT pathology. This book directs readers to the critical topics, highlights what an examiner regards as important core knowledge, and describes how best to structure answers when under pressure to perform. There are, however, benefits to reading this book at the beginning of training. For those just starting ENT training, it is difficult to know where to direct those first efforts which are currently dictated by departmental interests often without evidentiary basis. This book gives a succinct overview of what will be required over the years to come. It describes directed examination that is designed to diagnose. Examining a dizzy patient, for example, should not evoke horror but a growing confidence built on perfecting technique. To achieve their goal, Joseph and Peter have brought together colleagues from around the UK who have also recently excelled in the FRCS (ORL-HNS) examination. They bring a personal and up-to-date perspective on the examination, sharing their experience and tips. Senior editors who are at the top of our profession bring further insight into key topics that require particular attention.

In the following chapters you will learn all you need to know about how to pass the FRCS (ORL-HNS) examination. Examination skills and viva strategies are key components to making the grade. You'll learn model answers, pearls of wisdom, essential checklists in 'must-know' areas and pointers for further reading. *Advanced ENT Training: A Guide to Passing the FRCS (ORL-HNS) Examination* is a concise book designed to structure your learning in the most effective way. I therefore encourage you to read what will become the most important first and last book a trainee will read.

Patrick Axon, MBChB MD FRCS (ORL-HNS)
Consultant Otologist and Skull Base Surgeon
Cambridge University Hospitals

Editors

Joseph Manjaly is a consultant ENT surgeon at the Royal National ENT Hospital and University College London Hospitals, specialising in otology and auditory implant surgery. He completed higher surgical training in the London North Thames region and subsequently undertook a fellowship in otology and hearing implantation at Cambridge University Hospitals. He has held an interest in teaching since his undergraduate years at Bristol University and co-authored the first edition of the MasterPass book *ENT OSCEs: A Guide to Passing the DO-HNS and MRCS (ENT) OSCE* with Peter Kullar whilst a core trainee in Wessex Deanery. He has been actively involved in training issues regionally and nationally, holding a number of committee roles within the Association of Otolaryngologists in Training. In addition to being a keen sports fan he is also a musician who performs semi-professionally around the country with a band.

Peter Kullar is an NIHR clinical lecturer at Cambridge University Hospitals, having previously been a Wellcome Trust Clinical Research Fellow and academic ENT trainee in the Northern Deanery. He graduated from Cambridge University and subsequently completed a PhD from the same institution where his work elucidated mechanisms of mitochondrial-associated hearing loss. Peter co-authored the MasterPass book *ENT OSCEs: A Guide to Passing the DO-HNS and MRCS (ENT) OSCE* with Joseph Manjaly after they met during a course and concurred that there was a need for such a book amongst ENT trainees. Peter has held an active role in teaching and maintains a number of research streams with a specialist interest in otology.

Senior Section Editors

Manohar Bance, MBChB, MSc, FRCSC, FRCS, ABOto
Professor of Otology and Skull Base Surgery
University of Cambridge

and

Honorary Consultant
Cambridge University NHS Foundation Hospitals Trust
Cambridge, United Kingdom

Neil Donnelly, MBBS, MSc, FRCS (ORL-HNS)
Consultant ENT and Skull Base Surgeon
Cambridge University Hospitals
Cambridge, United Kingdom

Benjamin Hartley, FRCS
Consultant Paediatric Otolaryngologist
Great Ormond Street Hospital for Children
London, United Kingdom

Richard J Hewitt, BSc, FRCS (ORL-HNS)
Consultant Paediatric ENT, Head and Neck and Tracheal Surgeon
Great Ormond Street Hospital for Children
London, United Kingdom

James O'Hara, FRCS (ORL-HNS)
Consultant Otolaryngologist, Head and Neck Surgeon
The Freeman Hospital
Honorary Senior Clinical Lecturer
Newcastle University
Newcastle upon Tyne, United Kingdom

Hesham Saleh, FRCS (ORL-HNS)
Consultant Rhinologist/Facial Plastic Surgeon
Charing Cross and Royal Brompton Hospitals
Imperial College London
London, United Kingdom

James R Tysome, MA, PhD, FRCS (ORL-HNS)
Consultant ENT and Skull Base Surgeon
Cambridge University Hospitals
Cambridge, United Kingdom

Contributors

Chadwan Al-Yaghchi, MD, PhD, FRCS
(ORL-HNS)
Consultant ENT Surgeon
Imperial College Healthcare NHS Trust
London, United Kingdom

Nikul Amin, FRCS (ORL-HNS)
ENT Specialty Registrar
London Deanery – South
London, United Kingdom

Mohiemen Anwar, MBBS, PhD, FRCS
(ORL-HNS)
Consultant ENT Surgeon
Chelsea and Westminster NHS Foundation
Trust
London, United Kingdom

Jessica Bewick, MA, FRCS (ORL-HNS)
Consultant Paediatric ENT Surgeon
Cambridge University Hospitals NHS Trust
Cambridge, United Kingdom

Colin Butler, PhD, FRCS (ORL-HNS)
Paediatric ENT Fellow
Great Ormond Street Hospital for Children
London, United Kingdom

Alison Carter, BMedSci(Hons), BMBS,
DOHNS, FRCS (ORL-HNS)
ENT Specialty Registrar
London Deanery – North
London, United Kingdom

Nicholas Dawe, FRCSEd (ORL-HNS), MRes,
DipMedEd
Otology and Lateral Skull Base Fellow
Queen Elizabeth Hospital
University Hospitals Birmingham
Birmingham, United Kingdom

Susan Eitutis, BSc, MSc, MCISc
Research Audiologist
Emmeline Centre for Hearing Implants
Cambridge University Hospitals NHS Trust
Cambridge, United Kingdom

Matthew Ellis, MBBS, MPhil, FRCS
(ORL-HNS)
ENT Specialty Registrar
Northern Region
London Deanery – North
London, United Kingdom

Mark Ferguson, PhD, FRCS (ORL-HNS)
Royal College of Surgeons of England
Rhinology Fellow
Imperial College Healthcare NHS Trust
London, United Kingdom

Jason Fleming, MBBS Med, FRCS (ORL-HNS),
PhD
Head and Neck Fellow
University of Alabama
Birmingham, Alabama

Thomas Jacques, MA (Cantab), FRCS
(ORL-HNS)
ENT Specialty Registrar
London Deanery – North
London, United Kingdom

Kiran Jumani, MS (ENT), DNB
(Otolaryngology), FRCS (ORL-HNS)
Consultant ENT Surgeon
County Durham and Darlington NHS
Foundation Trust
Darlington, United Kingdom

Zi-Wei Liu, MBBS, FRCS (ORL-HNS)
ENT Specialty Registrar
London Deanery – North
London, United Kingdom

Gareth Lloyd, BMBS, BMedSci(Hons), FRCS
(ORL-HNS)
ENT Specialty Registrar
London Deanery – South
London, United Kingdom

Nishchay Mehta, PhD, FRCS (ORL-HNS)
ENT Specialty Registrar
London Deanery – North
London, United Kingdom

Jameel Muzaffar, BA (Hons), MBBS (Hons), MSc, FRCS (ORL-HNS)
ENT Specialty Registrar and Research Fellow/ PhD Student
Department of Clinical Neurosciences
University of Cambridge
Cambridge, United Kingdom

and

Academic Department of Military Surgery and Trauma
Royal Centre for Defence Medicine
University Hospitals Birmingham NHS Foundation Trust
Birmingham, United Kingdom

Robert Nash, MA(Oxon), DOHNS, FRCS (ORL-HNS), MA (KCL)
Consultant Otologist and Cochlear Implant Surgeon
Great Ormond Street Hospital for Children
London, United Kingdom

Lakhbinder Pabla, BMBCh MA (Oxon), DOHNS, FRCS (ORL-HNS), PGDipMedEd
Paediatric ENT Fellow
The Royal Children's Hospital
Melbourne, Australia

Eyal Schechter
Otology and Cochlear implant fellow
Addenbrooke's Hospital
Cambridge, United Kingdom

Sunil Sharma, MBBS, BSc (Hons), FRCS (ORL-HNS)
Consultant Paediatric ENT Surgeon
Alder Hey Children's NHS Foundation Trust
Liverpool, United Kingdom

Samit Unadkat, FRCS (ORL-HNS)
ENT Specialty Registrar
London Deanery – North
London, United Kingdom

Ananth Vijendren, BM, FRCS (ORL-HNS), PhD
Regional Otology and Implant Fellow
Cambridge University Hospitals NHS Trust
Cambridge, United Kingdom

Jagdeep Virk, MA, FRCS (ORL-HNS), PGCertMedEd
Head and Neck Fellow
Imperial College Healthcare NHS Trust
London, United Kingdom

Laura Warner, FRCS (ORL-HNS)
Consultant ENT Surgeon
The Newcastle upon Tyne Hospitals NHS Trust
Newcastle upon Tyne, United Kingdom

Abbreviations

A&E	accident and emergency
AABR	automated auditory brainstem response
ABC	airway, breathing, circulation
ABR	auditory brainstem response
ACC	adenoid cystic carcinoma
ACE	angiotensin-converting enzyme
ACP	antrochoanal polyp
AHI	apnoea–hypopnoea index
AICA	anterior inferior cerebellar artery
AJCC	American Joint Committee on Cancer
ANCA	antineutrophil cytoplasmic antibody
ARCP	Annual Review of Competence Progression
ARIA	allergic rhinitis and its impact on asthma
ATLS	Advanced Trauma Life Support
AVM	arteriovenous malformation
BAHA	bone-anchored hearing aid
BC	bone conduction
BCC	basal cell carcinoma
BDD	body dysmorphic disorder
BiCROS	bilateral contralateral routing of signal
BIH	benign intracranial hypertension
BMI	body mass index
BPPV	benign paroxysmal positional vertigo
BSACI	British Society for Allergy & Clinical Immunology
CBT	cognitive behavioural therapy
CMV	cytomegalovirus
CN	cranial nerve
CNS	central nervous system
COWS	cold opposite, warm same
CPA	cerebellopontine angle
CPAP	continuous positive airway pressure
CROS	contralateral routing of signal
CRP	C-reactive protein
CRS	chronic rhinosinusitis
CRT	chemoradiotherapy
CSOM	chronic suppurative otitis media
CT	computed tomography
cVEMP	cervical vestibular-evoked myogenic potential
CWD	canal-wall-down
CWU	canal-wall-up
CXR	chest X-ray
DVLA	Driver and Vehicle Licensing Agency
DVT	deep vein thrombosis
dW	diffusion-weighted
EAC	external auditory canal
EBER	Epstein–Barr small non-coding RNAs
EBV	Epstein–Barr virus
ECS	extracapsular spread

eGFR	estimated glomerular filtration rate
EMG	electromyography
ENG	electronystagmography
ENoG	electroneuronography
ENT	ears, nose and throat
EPOS	European Position Paper on Rhinosinusitis and Nasal Polyps
ESR	erythrocyte sedimentation rate
ET	endotracheal
ETT	endotracheal tube
EUA	examination under anaesthesia
FBC	full blood count
FDG-PET	fluorodeoxyglucose-positron emission tomography
FEES	fibreoptic endoscopic evaluation of swallowing
FESS	functional endoscopic sinus surgery
FLAIR	fluid attenuation inversion recovery
FNA	fine-needle aspiration
FNA-c	fine-needle aspiration cytology
FRCS (ORL-HNS)	Fellowship of the Royal College of Surgeons Otolaryngology – Head and Neck Surgery
FRCS	Fellowship of the Royal Colleges of Surgeons
GABHS	Group A beta-haemolytic Streptococcus
GCS	Glasgow Coma Scale
GORD	gastro-oesophageal reflux disease
GOSH	Great Ormond Street Hospital
GP	general practitioner
GPA	granulomatous polyangiitis
HB	House–Brackmann
HDU	high-dependency unit
HIV	human immunodeficiency virus
HNSCC	head and neck squamous cell carcinoma
HSV-1	herpes simplex virus-1
HZV	herpes zoster vaccine
IAC	internal auditory canal
ICA	internal carotid artery
ICON-S	International Collaboration on Oropharyngeal Cancer Network for Staging
ICP	intracranial pressure
IgE	immunoglobulin E
IJV	internal jugular vein
IMI	Institute of Medical Illustrators
IMRT	intensity-modulated radiotherapy
IMAX	internal maxillary artery
IOOG	International Otology Outcome Group
IT	intratympanic
ITU	intensive treatment unit
JCIE	Joint Committee on Intercollegiate Examinations
KTP	potassium-titanyl-phosphate
LA	local anaesthetic
LLC	lower lateral cartilage
LMA	laryngeal mask airway

MACH-NC	meta-analysis of chemotherapy in head and neck cancer
MACIS	metastases, age, complete surgery, invasion, size
MCT	medium-chain triglyceride
MDADI	MD Anderson Dysphagia Inventory
MdDS	mal de debarquement syndrome
MDT	multidisciplinary team
MEI	middle ear implant
MIBG	meta-iodobenzylguanidine
MR	magnetic resonance
MRA	magnetic resonance angiography
MRCS	Membership of the Royal Colleges of Surgeons
MRND	modified radical neck dissection
MS	multiple sclerosis
MUA	manipulation under anaesthesia
NG	nasogastric
NHS	National Health Service
NHSP	Newborn Hearing Screening Programme
NICU	newborn intensive care unit
NIHL	noise-induced hearing loss
non-EPI dwMRI	non-echo planar diffusion-weighted magnetic resonance imaging
NPC	nasopharyngeal carcinoma
NSAID	nonsteroidal anti-inflammatory drugs
OAE	otoacoustic emissions
OME	otitis media with effusion
ORN	osteoradionecrosis
OSA	obstructive sleep apnoea
PATHOS	post-operative adjuvant treatment for HPV-positive tumours
PC-BPPV	posterior canal BPPV
PCD	primary ciliary dyskinesia
PDA	patent ductus arteriosus
PEG	percutaneous endoscopic gastrostomy
PET-CT	positron emission tomography–computed tomography
PICA	posterior inferior cerebellar artery
PORP	partial ossicular replacement prosthesis
PORT	post-operative radiotherapy
PPIs	proton pump inhibitors
PPPD	persistent postural-perceptual dizziness
PTH	parathyroid hormone
RA	rheumatoid arthritis
RAI	radioactive iodine
RCT	randomised-controlled trial
RND	radical neck dissection
RRP	recurrent respiratory papillomatosis
RSTLs	relaxed skin tension lines
RT	radiotherapy
SCBU	special care baby unit
SCC	squamous cell carcinoma
SCIT	subcutaneous immunotherapy
SCM	sternocleidomastoid muscle

SH	social history
SLE	systemic lupus erythematosus
SLIT	sublingual immunotherapy
SLT	speech and language therapy
SMAS	superficial muscular aponeurotic system
SMG	submandibular gland
SND	selective neck dissection
SNHL	sensorineural hearing loss
SNUC	sinonasal undifferentiated carcinoma
SOAL	swallowing outcomes after laryngectomy
SPA	sphenopalatine artery
SPECT	single-photon emission computed tomography
SSNHL	sudden sensorineural hearing loss
SSQ	Sydney Swallow Questionnaire
SUV	standardised uptake value
TFTs	thyroid function tests
TM	tympanic membrane
TMJ	temporomandibular joint
TNM	tumour/node/metastasis
TORP	total ossicular replacement prosthesis
UICC	Union for International Cancer Control
ULC	upper lateral cartilage
UPSIT	University of Pennsylvania Smell Identification Test
URTI	upper respiratory tract infection
USS	ultrasound scan
VEGF	vascular endothelial growth factor
vHIT	video head impulse test
VNG	videonystagmography
VOG	video-oculography
VOR	vestibulo-ocular reflex
VPI	velopharyngeal insufficiency
VRA	visual reinforcement audiometry
WCC	white cell count
WHO	World Health Organisation

INTRODUCTION

JOSEPH MANJALY AND PETER KULLAR

1

You may remember in the early years of your training looking up to senior registrars who had become Fellows of the Royal College of Surgeons, feeling that you had a long way to go before you had the knowledge and experience to join them. As you progress through training and the end of ST6 draws near, it's not unheard of to start developing imposter syndrome. Are you truly ready for this hurdle? Or have you somehow slipped under the radar because everyone has assumed that you were doing fine? Is everything about to suddenly hit the fan with an ignominious revelation that you eternally follow patients up in clinic and can only just about do a tracheostomy?

And yet the FRCS (ORL-HNS), just like other exams you have passed along the way, is a very passable exam. You've reached this point because you are capable of meeting that standard. Once you have done so the next step will be to think about a consultant post, usually within 18 months though that may seem a far-away idea at this point.

What has probably changed since your last exam are your circumstances. As a registrar the need to be on top form every day, particularly on operating days, limits the number of late nights you can reasonably spend revising. Gone are the string of post-nights 'zero days' you could use as a senior house officer. You may have family responsibilities to juggle by now. The tools to be able to 'work smart' are more crucial than ever and our book is written in this spirit.

The syllabus for this exam seems endless: essentially try and know everything about ENT and its related specialities. There are many excellent texts and resources available for the task but arguably the most useful information is the pragmatic, working knowledge and gems of wisdom handed down by the preceding generations. In this book we have tried to bring these together in one place.

More than just a question and answer book, we hope this book will act as a coaching manual. Every section is centred on a combination of '*model answers*', pearls of wisdom, checklists (✓) and pointers for further reading (✎). Rather than being an exhaustive ENT text, we hope this book will guide you to exam success in a thorough yet efficient manner alongside your work commitments. We have been comprehensive with topic selection. The viva topics included in this book touch on nearly every subject that has come up in the exam in the 5 years prior to publication.

We have gratefully called on contributions from colleagues around the country. All were identified as high achievers with a skill for teaching and mentoring. Thankfully for us, all have responded with enthusiasm and willingness to be a part of this project. All viva advice contributors have passed the exam within the last 3 years, including multiple gold medal winners. We are sure that many will go on to be leaders of their fields in the future.

The authority of this book is secured by our senior editors. In Manohar Bance, Neil Donnelly, Ben Hartley, Richard Hewitt, James O'Hara, Hesham Saleh and James Tysome, we have had the privilege of receiving internationally respected wisdom from current national and world-leading clinicians. We are very grateful for their time and critical input.

Preparing for the FRCS (ORL-HNS) examination will be a tough journey – both for you and those around you. We hope this book will help you prepare whether you're a UK or international trainee. It will be a time when your patient care significantly matures. Enjoy seeing the rewards of that. You may end up strangely wishing you had gone through the whole thing earlier!

PERSONAL REFLECTIONS ON THE FRCS (ORL-HNS) PART 1 EXPERIENCE

ALISON CARTER

2

Currently the earliest point in training to be eligible to sit the exam is the beginning of ST7. If you are in a training programme that allows you to pick your jobs for the next year, it is important to select carefully. Now may not be the time to rank the busiest job in the deanery or the one with the longest commute. I returned to a hospital at which I had worked previously, where my colleagues were supportive and understood that my main focus over the coming months was the exam.

I have summarised my approach to the exam but this of course is very individual.

Many of my successful colleagues approached things slightly differently, so it is worth talking to those around you and so you can synthesise a strategy that suits you best. I hope this guide will give you an idea of what worked for me and what may work for you.

6 Months Pre-exam

Applications will be via the JCIE website (www.jcie.org.uk) and require you to fill in an electronic form with your work history, dates of your MRCS and university medical degree, a summary of your operative experience (a PDF of your elogbook is sufficient), your curriculum vitae, and three structured references from supervisors whom you have worked with in the last 2 years. If you are in a UK training programme this must include one from your training programme director stating that you have a ST6 ARCP outcome 1. The referees are asked to assess your diagnostic skills, clinical management, operative skills, professionalism and probity and communication and language skills. Getting the forms signed always takes longer than one might anticipate so make sure that you are organised in getting this done.

At the point of application, you have to pay for both parts of the FRCS (at the time of writing: Part 1 – £536, Part 2 – £1,313, total £1,849). Most will elect to do Part 2 FRCS in the next available sitting on the application form (3–4 months post Part 1). There have been occasions where the second part has been oversubscribed and entry is granted in order of receipt of applications, therefore in order to avoid any unnecessary stress or disappointment later an early application is advised.

Over your training you have likely been building your CV with publications, quality improvement projections and further degrees, but now is time to put all that to one side. Accept that for the 3–4 months before the exam, you will not be doing any of those things, and try and use the 6-month mark before the Part 1 to finish outstanding projects so that you can start revising with a clean slate. I was surprised at how understanding my colleagues and bosses were about this when politely declining to take on any extra projects, and was usually met with 'of course, you have the exam – best of luck'.

4 Months Pre-exam

Gone are the days of university when you could dedicate hours on end to revision. You will likely be working in a busy job with long days, may have accumulated other things in your life such as partners and children and sadly dealing with sleep deprivation is probably not as easy as it once was all those years ago. Remind yourself that most people sitting the exam are also facing the same challenges, and you just have to manage it as best you can.

Look at your work week and try and identify areas where you can get some productive revision time in. You may have a morning or afternoon in your timetable that can be used for revision. Be disciplined in making sure that you use it effectively. Work out when you are at your most productive. For me, I know that I work better in the morning, and on looking at my timetable, three mornings I had to be at work for 7.30 a.m., but the other two were 9 a.m. Although it required a lot of dedication, and some that the alarm was switched off for, for those 2 days a week, I would wake up at 5.30 a.m. and get 2–3 hours done before work. In return, I never revised in the evenings, and made sure that I enjoyed times out with friends or relaxing at home 'guilt free'. Although this worked for me, I know that not everyone would work best in the mornings, so be honest with yourself as to what your golden hours are, make it happen and make sure you enjoy the other hours and give yourself a break. At the weekend I had one day where I was productive (sometimes both), but again never worked in the evenings.

I started my revision using a textbook to give an overview of all the areas of ENT. I read through topic by topic, highlighting things I thought were important. Everyone responds differently to different styles of books, and I would recommend asking your colleagues what they found helpful previously and going to look at a few of them in the library or sample them online, before buying one which you think you will like. You do not need a book that goes into intricate detail, this is more for an overview of different topics, some of which you may not have had as much exposure to in your training, and to jog your memory on those you have. Although most of the FRCS courses are aimed at Part 2, there are some available for Part 1 and can help refining exam technique and identify gaps in your knowledge.

It can also be good to think of something else other than your exams, such as a holiday to look forward to, or perhaps a challenge to focus on training for a half marathon, enabling you to break up your revision.

2 Months Pre-exam

I started to look at some example questions in the various books available (although some of my colleagues did start this earlier alongside their reading). Some of the books available had explanations attached to the answers so I used those ones preferentially as it is a good way to continue your revision and to learn from your answers. If there was an area where I had not got it right, or I thought it was a good 'fact', I wrote it down in my notes.

1 Month Pre-exam

Try and take some time off work before the exam. For me, this was December, and being around Christmas, there were natural days off work which were helpful, and I did not have to take that many days off surrounding them to take 2 weeks off prior to the exam, with a few interspersed on calls. I kept my format the same, waking up and getting straight to work, and then using my evenings to relax and put my laptop and books away.

1 Week Pre-exam

I typed up all my notes at the beginning of the week that I had made and then tried to reread them on top of continuing to do questions. This was a hard week as you are exhausted and you feel like nothing is going in, in fact you feel that knowledge is somehow being pushed out by anything new you learn and that you are now destined for failure. It is hard to trust in the work that you have done, but the fear of having to do the exam again if I failed helped to focus me over the last few days.

On the Day

Part 1 is done at local professional testing centres, where they were very formal about the exam. All you are required to bring is your photo ID. You may take the exam sitting in a room with others taking completely different exams. The only other items offered were tissues and earplugs, which they provide. It is computer based and very self-explanatory on how it worked with moving between questions. There is the ability to flag questions for review later on, and before finishing the exam it tells you if you had any question that you did not answer (there is no negative marking so you should attempt all questions). There are laminate sheets with marker pens available for making notes which you are not allowed to take out after. The first paper was single best answer (2 hours) and then there was a 1-hour lunch break when we were allowed to leave, and then return for the extended matching questions (2.5 hours). Results usually arrive within 4 weeks.

So Where Do You Start?

Part 1 of the FRCS is designed to test breadth, so it is impossible to give a discrete list of topics to study. On the day of the exam you will no doubt feel that some of the topics were niche and perhaps not what you would see in your 'day to day' of ENT clinics and theatres. The following are examples of topics that have been asked previously, purely to give a flavour of the breadth required and the overlap with other related medical specialties.

Paediatrics: Syndromes affecting hearing/smell/facial features/swallowing/airway, neck masses.

Rhinology: Nasal masses, hereditary haemorrhagic telangiectasia, disorders of smell, acoustic rhinometry/rhinomanometry.

Facial plastics and reconstruction: Pinnaplasty, rhinoplasty types, reconstructive flaps, skin cancer types and treatment.

Head and neck: Neck dissection types, radiotherapy RT/chemotherapy, swallowing physiology and disorders, oral lesions, parapharyngeal masses and infections, OSA, vocal cord anatomy, TNM and staging for each type of head and neck cancer and salivary disease.

Otology: External ear masses, cholesteatoma theories, complications of acute otitis media, inner ear malformations, nystagmus types and causes.

Trauma and emergency management: GCS, Le Fort fractures, paediatric and adult resuscitation, shock treatment, neck trauma, imbalance of electrolytes with their ECG changes, symptoms and management.

Pharmacology: LA types, doses and duration of action, otological drop contents, nasal medication contents, vestibular medication, migraine medication and antibiotic types.

Radiology: CT and MRI for different pathologies, different sequences and appearance of anatomy and what they are used for.

Audiology: Paediatric testing, ABRs, hearing loss types, presbyacusis subtypes, vestibular testing and hearing aid types.

Anatomy: Skull base, sinuses, middle ear, facial nerve pathway and sections, lymphatic drainage pathways, CN anatomy and referred pain anatomical pathways.

Research: Levels of evidence, statistical tests.

Basic sciences: Bacteria and viruses relevant to ENT, inflammatory response/mediators, autoantibodies, autoimmune disease, embryology e.g. branchial arch/cleft/pouch derivatives, patterns of inheritance, coagulation pathways, cell genetics and tumour genes.

Miscellaneous: Migraine types, vestibular disorders, LASER types and uses and examination signs relevant to ENT.

Essentially, try and keep your revision broad. Do as many practice questions as you can find. The examination is marked in such a way that questions with a high variance in candidates' answers may be discarded, but you should aim to know the facts that all your colleagues know.

GENERAL ADVICE FOR PREPARING FOR PART 2

JOSEPH MANJALY

3

With Part 1 results generally taking 3–4 weeks to arrive, you will typically have a minimum of 2–3 months to prepare for Part 2. Although it doesn't feel like it, this will be enough time and it seems sensible to allow a break between the two exams. The exam runs over 3 days, though you will only be required for 2 consecutive days. The location rotates around the UK and Ireland twice a year. One of your exam days will consist of four 30-minute vivas, usually in a hotel. Your other day is based in hospital with two 30-minute clinical stations (two patients per station) and a separate communication skills station. Once you know the exam dates and location, book yourself a hotel room and travel arrangements. Nearly everyone books into the hotel in which the vivas are taking place. I would recommend this – it minimises any travel issues on the day and you can be around others as much or as little as you wish. There is a lot of waiting between stations and I personally found it helpful to have company.

Courses for Part 2 are a good idea. There are plenty advertised all over the country and going on one or two is helpful midway through your preparation. The difference between factual knowledge and exam technique will become clear and it's also a good chance to mix with candidates outside your own region. This brings me to the most significant piece of advice: be a team player. Revising in groups is crucial for Part 2. This is not an exam to learn alone purely from books. I regularly met up with five others from my region, at least once a week in the 8 weeks leading up to the exam. We gave each other practice questions and feedback. Crucially we made a commitment to sincerely try and improve each other with honest feedback and passing on inherited tips. Whenever any of us arranged viva practice with consultants in the region, we would organise it so that the whole group could come. We used group messaging regularly for both parts of the exam and shared a communal cloud storage drive for all our articles, topic lists and practice questions. Video conferencing apps are a great way to exchange practice questions with trainees from other regions and gain a different perspective. When fatigue set in, I found it particularly motivating being part of five-way online question practice session – most of all for the reassurance that you're on the right track compared with everyone else.

Finally, arrange plenty of practice sessions with consultants in your region. There is a lot of good will out there to help get you through. These sessions were really valuable for bringing into focus some of the topics that you may not have had a lot of direct exposure to in your training. Don't forget to keep track of whom to share your good news with when you pass!

Advice for Part 2 Vivas

Your four 30-minute vivas will be spread across a whole day. Decide how you will prefer to spend the very long gaps in between. Each session covers one of the four subspecialties (head and neck, otology, rhinology and facial plastics, paediatric ENT). Within each you will typically have six 5-minute topics. The vivas all take place in one large hall with around 20 candidates being examined at a time – lots of background noise! At each station you will sit opposite the two examiners who usually take it in turn to ask questions whilst the other takes notes.

Five minutes per topic passes very quickly and it is important to succinctly respond to the initial question to move the examiners on to more challenging areas. The initial question will typically be designed to get you going e.g. describe this photograph; explain how you would assess a patient with a 2-year history of swallowing difficulties; describe this audiogram, etc. This may then lead onto a more pass/fail level question before the examiners have the freedom to push you in different areas for higher marks. Be prepared to draw if asked. You will read that quoting key papers and classifications is needed to score top marks, however, the questions are rarely designed to allow for this. The key is to do the basics well but relatively quickly, showing clear and sensible reasoning before demonstrating the ability to handle more niche areas. Be wary, your desire to steer a conversation towards a specific journal article must not distract you from being comprehensive with the initial questioning where the majority of marks will be scored.

For example, when questioned on a child who has failed ABR testing during neonatal hearing screening, one could be armed with every last detail on the further subjective, objective, genetic and radiological tests – but if you fail to suggest initially that the first step is to refer to paediatric audiology and repeat the ABR, the examiner may not even let you advance to the next question! Five minutes can pass very quickly.

If you reach a point in any viva where you are stuck, try and at least express your thought process logically. Aim to do this in a mature confident way, filling the shoes of a new consultant having a discussion with a senior colleague. Even for the best candidates some stations will go better than others. You may even do better in topics that you normally wouldn't favour. What's crucial is to be able to move on from a bad question. With so many different marking points across the exam, there are many opportunities to make up for one low score, but you can't afford to collapse in your first question of the 30-minute viva and consequently underperform on the other five. This is even more true of the clinical stations, where the potential to be humbled in front of your patient can be very off-putting.

Advice for Part 2 Clinical Stations

Another crucial piece of advice: The clinical stations are very much vivas in their own right, only with real patients rather than photographs. You will typically be asked to perform an observed history and/or specific examination with a genuine patient and this will be followed by several viva-style questions. This may include being asked to interpret radiological images. There is a temptation to spend all your Part 2 preparation practising vivas based on photographs and overlook this section. However, these are far more than just choreographed examination rituals and if this is forgotten candidates can easily be caught out.

You will have two 30-minute stations, taking place in hospital clinic rooms. In one station will be 15 minutes with an otology patient and 15 minutes with a head and neck patient. In the other will be 15 minutes of rhinology or facial plastics and 15 minutes of paediatric ENT (typically a child with a parent). You will have two examiners in the room with you. There may be further examiners observing. Each may move around you during examinations to see exactly what you are doing. You should be ready for this and not be unnerved!

Be ready to take a thorough history from a patient with any sort of ENT problem. Your examination technique must be rehearsed thoroughly so that you can perform them fluently. Listen carefully to what is asked though and if you are only asked to perform a specific portion of an examination (e.g. perform tuning fork tests) then do just that.

In junior-level exams performing the examination routine was all that was required. At this level you need to be able to confidently interpret and explain your findings to the examiner, in front of your patient. In reality this is exactly what you do in clinic all the time but doing it confidently in the exam setting is helped with some practice! Are you sure you can describe the post-operative ear? Are you absolutely confident those tuning fork tests are what you expected for this patient? Be prepared for patients who have had some form of historical, unrecognisable operation, for you now have to rapidly figure out what have been done and why they have these anatomical and functional abnormalities! Don't forget the alcohol gel. We were asked to bring our own headlight but in the end any piece of equipment we needed was provided.

These are abnormal scenarios disguised as normal scenarios. You may be asked to perform a seemingly simple examination and explain your findings with a patient for whom you have neither taken the history, nor importantly established rapport with. This can put you off your stride for example when describing someone's nose! Try and break the ice before you do anything else – introduce yourself with a smile, thank the patient for coming in today and perhaps ask them if they mind you speaking to the examiner about them. You will find your own particular version of this but putting yourself and the patient at ease makes a big difference to the rest of the encounter. This is even more true in the paediatric station with children and their parents. Have they found it tiring being asked the same questions by some many doctors in one day? Have they had a day off school? Remember that they are still patients. Remind them that you are a compassionate human being both inside and outside of the examination room – your examiners will appreciate it.

Advice for Part 2 Communication Skills

This station also takes place in a hospital clinic room and lasts 20 minutes with two examiners and an actor playing the role of a patient or family member. You will typically be given a written scenario to read prior to the encounter and the plot will usually consist of history taking, some time spent giving information back based on that history, and possibly a twist in the story – for example a scan that shows a cancer when your original conversation was about a benign condition.

You will be judged on your etiquette, rapport, verbal and non-verbal skills. Though not necessarily the focus of the assessment, you will still be required to exercise sensible clinical judgement and interpretation within the context of the scenario. Thoroughness, sympathy, safety-netting and MDT involvement should be remembered. If you can foresee a potential twist in the scenario then it may help to counsel the patient more thoroughly to begin with and soften any challenging emotions later in the conversation. Ultimately, if you do what you usually do in clinic – safely and thoroughly, with clear language and rapport, this station should not be an obstacle. Those for whom English isn't their first language perhaps may find it helpful to spend a little more preparation time on this station and seek feedback from mentors. The history and communication skills sections of our MasterPass series textbook '*ENT OSCEs*' are equally relevant for this part.

HISTORIES AND EXAMINATIONS IN THE PART 2 CLINICAL SECTION

JOSEPH MANJALY AND PETER KULLAR

4

The FRCS examination demands a fluent approach to the examination of the head and neck. You will have taken histories and performed ENT examinations on many hundreds of patients by the time you come to sit the exam. However, this means there may be an element of 'unlearning' shortcuts you have been practising over the years. You will need to adopt a comprehensive and systematic approach for examining ENT subsites that is easy to remember. You can then apply the appropriate routine swiftly and confidently so that you can spend more time focussing on how you will present your findings fluently and discuss your interpretation.

Basic schemes for these histories and examinations are covered thoroughly in our earlier publication *ENT OSCEs – A Guide to Passing the DO-HNS and MRCS (ENT) OSCE*. Though that book was designed for an exam you've already passed, the examination sections are appropriately thorough and equally applicable to this exam, so we will not aim to comprehensively cover those elements again here. Rather we will try and provide some guidance specific to the FRCS exam and focus on the advanced areas that trainees find more challenging.

As a starting point, revise your examination routines for ear, nose, neck, thyroid, parotid, oral cavity, CNs and balance.

There are a few general rules for the examination stations:

- Always introduce yourself and gain the patient's consent for examination.
- Ask if the patient currently has any pain.
- Remember to remain 'bare below the elbows' and use alcohol gel when provided.
- Be logical and confident despite the unusual context to this patient interaction. If it helps to establish rapport, ask the patient if they mind you talking about them to the examiner.

Ear Examination

- Unless instructed otherwise, offer to examine the better ear first.
- You are often asked to examine patients who have had previous surgery. Be sure to thoroughly inspect and feel the post-auricular and temporal region for pinna abnormalities, scars, pits, bone anchored hearing aid abutments and cochlear implant packages under the skin.
- Your inspection should then focus on:
  - Pinna (compare each side, scars, infections, piercings, quality of skin and cartilage). Specifically examining each subsite – helix, antihelix, tragus and conchal bowl
  - Mastoid (check by moving pinna forward, check skin quality and colour, signs of infection, post-auricular incisions)
  - Pre-auricular area (check for sinuses, fistulas, pits, endaural incision)

- It is worth having a microtia grading system in your mind to describe any pinna abnormalities (see the microtia chapter in the Paediatric ENT section of this book).
- Examine the EAC and TM using the otoscope. The speculum that gives the most complete view of the TM should be selected as the smaller the field of view the harder it is for you to mentally reconstruct an image of the entire TM.
- Comment specifically on:
  - EAC (discharge, bony swellings, erosions, cholesteatoma)
  - Pars tensa (perforations, atelectasis, retraction pockets, status of ossicles)
  - Pars flaccida (attic retraction pockets, cholesteatoma)
- Mastoid cavities are a very common finding at this point. Make sure you have a concise way of describing what you see: *'Evidence of a previous canal wall down mastoidectomy with a cavity that is dry and well epithelialised. The facial ridge is low and there is a wide meatoplasty'.*
- Mention to the examiner that it is also possible to perform pneumatic otoscopy to assess the movement of the TM (this can be simulated by asking the patient to perform the Valsalva manoeuvre).
- Perform the fistula test by applying pressure on the tragus. A positive test reveals nystagmus with the fast phase away from the fistula side.
- Perform free-field hearing test. This technique is important to master as reliable audiometry may not always be available. This test is used either as a screening method to determine whether a hearing loss is present in one or both ears and also as a method to define the level of hearing impairment.
- Explain to the patient that numbers and letters will be spoken or whispered and ask the patient to repeat them. The examiner should position themself behind the patient so that lip reading is not possible. Start the test by using a loud voice to say easily recognisable numbers such as '99', this ensures that the patient understands the test. Testing of each ear should be performed whilst masking the contralateral side (most easily done by occluding the EAC with the tragus whilst gently rubbing). It is routine to start by testing the better hearing ear first.
  - *Screening test*: If a patient cannot repeat back what is said in a whispered voice at 60 cm then they have a hearing impairment.
  - Next define the level of impairment by finding the patient's free-field threshold which is the voice level and distance at which they get more than 50% right.

Voice level	Distance (cm)	Threshold (dB)
Whisper	60	12
Whisper	10	34
Conversational voice	60	48
Conversational voice	10	56
Loud voice	60	76

- Perform Rinne and Weber tests to distinguish between sensorineural and conductive hearing loss using the 512-Hz fork.

- Patients with facial nerve palsies are common both here and in the head and neck station. The challenge is being able to examine the facial nerve swiftly whilst being able to interpret your findings in the context of the clinical scenario. You should ask the patient to raise eyebrows, close eyes tightly, wrinkle the nose, show their teeth and blow cheeks against resistance. The findings should be reported using the House–Brackmann classification.
- To complete the examination, state that you would like to examine the patient's ears under the microscope, complete the CN examination, examine the neck and also the post-nasal space as appropriate to the case.

Rhinology and Facial Plastics Examination

- Most often this entails a rhinoplasty assessment, however alternatives include the skin cancer assessment or a patient with nasal obstruction presented with a scan leading to a discussion on vasculitis or a sinonasal tumour. See all the relevant viva chapters for these conditions and have your examination routines and explanations well prepared.
- Assessment for rhinoplasty involves the examination of the patient, their face and of course their nose. Clarify from the examiner exactly what you're being asked to do. If in your history the patient discusses wishing to have a rhinoplasty it may be appropriate to explore motivations for surgery. Be aware of conditions such as body dysmorphic disorder (BDD) as rhinoplasty may compound rather than alleviate the patient's problems with body image.
- Assessment of the face includes thinking about symmetry and ethnicity.
- Inspect the skin of the nose, commenting on its thickness/thinness.
- Inspect the shape of the nose from the front:
  - Look for any breaks in the brow-tip line.
  - Look at the nasal width. The alar base should ideally be equal to the intercanthal distance.
  - Consider any visible deviations in terms of thirds.
  - Consider the nasal length. The distance from radix to tip should be similar to the distance from stomium to menton.
  - Look at the shape of the nasal tip. Be able to describe any asymmetry, bifidity, rotation and bulbosity. Assess the lateral crura of the LLC and look for any columellar show.
  - Examine the nose from above and below.
  - Palpate the nose to further examine the skin and tip recoil, as well as revealing any columellar dislocation.
- Inspect the nose from the side:
  - It may or may not be practical in the exam to recite and interpret every available angle, but it is useful to have an understanding of the different elements in case specifically asked. Here is a list of points to consider:
    - The Frankfort line (cephalic tragus to infra-orbital rim), which should be perpendicular to the facial line (glabellar to chin)
    - Nasal projection, calculated as a ratio of the tip-alar distance over the tip-nasion distance, ideally being around 0.6 (Goode's ratio)
    - Nasofrontal angle (115°–135°)

- Nasofacial angle (30°–40°)
- Nasomental angle (120°–132°)
- Mentocervical angle (80°–95°) (Figure 4.1)
  - Be able to describe abnormalities of the nasal dorsum, such as a hump and saddling.
- When assessing nasal obstruction, have a systematic approach to anterior rhinoscopy.
- Understand the functional importance of the nasal valve areas. The external nasal valve is bounded by the caudal edge of the LLC and the nasal alae. The internal valve is bounded by the inferior turbinate, pyriform aperture, nasal septum and caudal edge of the ULC. The internal nasal valve angle is between the ULC and the septum (normally 10°–15°).

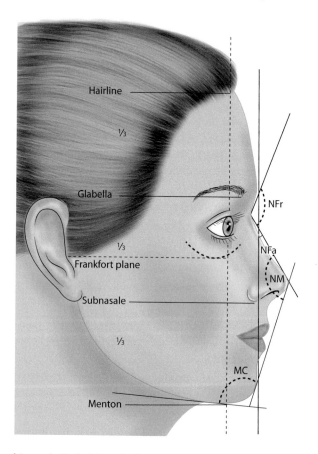

Figure 4.1   Angles used in aesthetic facial analysis.

Advice for Examining the Oral Cavity, Neck, Thyroid and Parotid Glands

- These examinations are covered comprehensively in *ENT OSCEs – A Guide to Passing the DO-HNS and MRCS (ENT) OSCE*.
- Be particularly prepared for patients with thyroid lumps and thyroglossal cysts who are often well and easy to find for exams. Be well versed in discussing the investigation and management of such pathologies.

- Other neck lumps may well appear here and the relevant viva chapters in this book will help with these. Often you will be faced with a previously operated patient who may have scars to find and CN pathology.
- Be able to describe different neck scars, the likely operation, and think which structures may be removed as part of this surgery performed.
- Primary parotid lesions may appear in this station. Remember that the parotid can be the site of secondary lesions from skin cancers that have required parotid surgery with a resulting facial palsy.
- This would also be an appropriate station to be faced with questions around tracheostomy and laryngectomy care.

Advice for Examining a Child in the Paediatric Examination

- Of course, an important part of this examination is your rapport with both the parent and the child and maintaining a comfortable pain-free interaction.
- A variety of different clinical scenarios can occur here, relevant to otology, rhinology and head and neck.
- Be well prepared for cases of chronic otitis media, glue ear and OSA. Prominent ears would also be a fair topic here.
- Branchial anomalies often feature. Look out for second branchial cleft fistulas and pre-auricular sinuses and remember to complete your examination with any underlying syndrome in mind.
- One area you will almost certainly need to prepare is a system for examining a child with classical syndromic features. See the viva chapter on syndromes in ENT and be able to recognise and describe the features of all the syndromes included. A systematic examination would include an overall assessment of the child followed by specific assessment of face (including eyes), facial nerve, neck (tracheostomy and scars), ears and hearing implants, mouth, tongue and jaw and finally enquiring about any other systemic features and feeding routes.

Advice for Undertaking an Examination of Balance

- This is an area most trainees fear and find most difficult to interpret, so we have intentionally dedicated more book space to this topic. It is unlikely you will be asked to perform a comprehensive vestibular assessment with follow up questions in 15 minutes. However, it would be very reasonable to ask a trainee to perform certain elements of the assessment dependent on the patient's history and follow this up with specific questions. Don't get caught out!

To explain everything you might possibly need to know for this part of the exam, we have asked Professor Manohar Bance to detail his systematic approach to the vestibular assessment.

Examining the 'Dizzy' Patient

MANOHAR BANCE

The neurotologic exam for vertiginous and balance conditions can conceptually be divided into tests that:

1. *Test for a fixed lesion in the vestibular system* (including unmasking a lesion that has been compensated for). Examples are the sudden head-thrust test and post head-shake nystagmus.
2. *Provoke excitable vestibular reactivity*, such as Dix–Hallpike positioning.
3. *Exclude serious neurologic pathology*, such as CN or cerebellar testing.
4. *Test balance dysfunction*, which can be central or peripheral in origin, such as Unterberger's stepping test or joint position testing.

Consider the examination in sections:

The first step is always to take a step back and look at the general patient profile.

> Are there syndromic features? Is there a facial paralysis to suggest a temporal bone lesion? Is there a head tilt (acute uncompensated vestibular loss or cerebellar lesion), a Horner's syndrome (brainstem pathology), etc. This step can be forgotten but is important.

Tests are classified into six main testing categories. Whether to do special vestibular tests such as fistula testing is guided by a history suggesting specific pathologies.

1. Oculomotor testing
2. Vestibular testing
3. Balance and gait testing
4. CN exam
5. Cerebellar testing
6. Special tests that depend on the history

Oculomotor testing

Oculomotor testing is a good section to start with, as it is relatively non-threatening, and builds rapport.

Nystagmus

Start by looking for primary or gaze-evoked nystagmus.

Nystagmus in the primary position (i.e. eyes looking forward in the centre of the eye socket) can be horizontal, oblique, vertical or torsional, or it can be a mixture such as pendular nystagmus, which is usually congenital. If nystagmus is present with visual fixation, it is always abnormal.

The most likely vestibular evoked nystagmus will be horizontal or horizontal-torsional, as this arises from an acute vestibular loss. The fast phase of the nystagmus beats towards the 'good' ear. If it is peripheral in origin, it should:

- Get worse when looking towards the fast phase (Alexander's law)
- Be conjugate (i.e. both eyes move exactly together)
- Be direction fixed (i.e. always beats in the same direction regardless of eye position)
- Suppressed by fixation, although this cannot be tested clinically easily unless Frenzel's lenses are provided.

Next ask the patient to look left, right, up and down to look for gaze-evoked conditions. Eye excursions should be only to the punctum of the lower lacrimal duct (about 30°) as past this you may provoke physiologic nystagmus. Physiologic nystagmus settles after a few beats.

This may elicit 'gaze-evoked' nystagmus. Gaze-evoked nystagmus can be vestibular i.e. direction fixed and with a 'sawtooth' or 'jerk' pattern (Figure 4.2a), or central in origin.

(a)   (b)

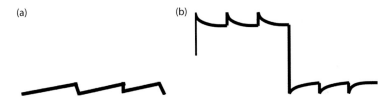

Figure 4.2   (a) Up is right, down is left, this is left-beating vestibular nystagmus. (b) Up is right, down is left, this is direction changing gaze-evoked, coarse nystagmus.

If the nystagmus only comes on with lateral gaze to one side, it could be the last stage of a compensating vestibular nystagmus i.e. only coming on when looking towards the good ear (grade 1 nystagmus). Other type of gaze-evoked nystagmus is a coarser 'saddle-shaped' nystagmus (Figure 4.2b) which is caused by the loss of the central brainstem neural integrator which keeps the eyes eccentrically placed once they are brought there. This is often bidirectional and direction changing i.e. left beating on left gaze, and right beating on right gaze.

A special type of nystagmus is the one that is 'jerk' type to one side and coarser gaze-evoked type to the other side. For example a 'jerk' pattern beating to left on looking left and a coarse 'saddle-shaped' pattern on looking right, this is called Brun nystagmus, and is due to a large lesion in the CPA, most often a vestibular schwannoma (on the side of the coarse nystagmus).

Upbeat and downbeat nystagmus also follow Alexander's law and are central in origin (e.g. Arnold-Chiari, MS, stroke and drugs).

Smooth ocular pursuit

Ask the patient to follow your finger from side to side, making an excursion of about 30° to each side, at about 0.5 Hz. Young healthy subjects should be able to follow this very smoothly with their eyes. Good instruction is important e.g. 'follow my finger very carefully with your eyes and try to keep your eyes completely on it when it is moving'. Even if there is only a short segment of good smooth pursuit, this is normal, some patients make repeated saccades away from the target.

Abnormal smooth pursuit means the patient cannot follow smoothly and uses a series of saccades to stay on track (Figure 4.3), called 'saccadic smooth pursuit'. This can be normal in much older subjects, and can also occur due to some drugs such as anticonvulsants. While it is not very localising in the brain, very saccadic smooth pursuit usually occurs with brainstem or cerebellar lesions.

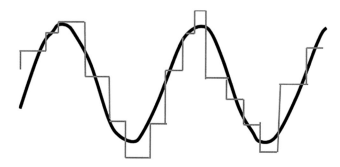

Figure 4.3   Saccadic smooth pursuit. Black is the target position and brown is the eye position.

Saccadic testing

Ask the subject to look at from one finger to the other, placed about 60° apart on either side of the mid-line (there are more sophisticated tests but this is the most practical). The patient should be able to make eye movements cleanly from one finger to the other. It is acceptable to make a large saccade and then a small 'micro-saccade' to acquire the target, but it is always abnormal to overshoot the target and make a saccade to get back to it, or to stop short of the target and then see the eye glide towards the target (glissade).

This usually indicates serious brainstem or cerebellar pathology if present. Saccadic abnormalities are rarer. Saccades can also be tested in the vertical plane. Be careful of micro-saccadic oscillations, some patients make very small saccades all the time, even when asked to look at a target, and these are not always associated with any serious central pathology.

Vestibular testing

Vestibular testing in the clinical exam is only really practical for the *lateral semicircular canal.* The main test that would be expected is the **head-impulse test** (also called the Halmagyi head thrust).

Start by asking the patient if they have any neck problems, as this test can be uncomfortable if there are. The head should be turned to one side about 30°–40°, and the patient asked to fixate on the examiner's nose and stay on it during the head thrust. The head is then rapidly rotated to the mid-line. In a normal head thrust, the eyes do not move at all during and after the head movement.

If there is a lesion (on the side the head is moving TOWARDs i.e. turned to left and rapidly rotated to right to reach mid-line, then testing right ear, and vice versa), then the eyes do not sufficiently counter-roll with the VOR and undershoot the target, and a small saccade is made to the target (nose). This eye movement can be hard to see, and the test may have to be repeated. It's important to make the head thrust unpredictable, otherwise the patient may make a 'covert' saccade in the middle of the neck turn and end up on target without using their VOR. This is a test of the high-frequency function of the lateral canal, and usually requires a substantial amount of vestibular loss to be positive.

Another test that can 'unmask' a compensated vestibular loss is the **post head-shake nystagmus test.**

In this test (usually under Frenzel's lenses) the head is shaken side to side for about 30 seconds at 1 Hz.

After stopping, a positive test is the onset of nystagmus that beats towards the good ear. It can be biphasic (i.e. change direction after several seconds), or even triphasic, but these types are uncommon.

Gait tests

These tests are for testing vestibulo-spinal function, cerebellar function and proprioceptive function. Most are normal or only subtly abnormal in compensated vestibular loss.

However, in acute vestibular loss, bilateral vestibular loss or in central lesions, there may be marked imbalance. There are many gait tests, from **Romberg's** (standing with eyes closed) to heel-toe walking, standing on one foot, sit to stand, etc., but the most common one is **Unterberger's stepping (or Fukuda) test.**

The patient is asked to step in place for about a minute (about 50–60 steps) with eyes closed and both arms raised at 90° in front of them. It is important they raise their legs adequately i.e. actually march on the spot (Figure 4.4).

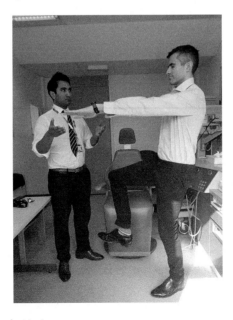

Figure 4.4   Unterberger's stepping test.

A rotation of more than 30° to one side (classically towards the vestibular weak side) is considered abnormal. However, the test is not reliable, and it is more important to look for stumbling, or gross imbalance during the test than rotation. This indicates some problem with gait control, which may be vestibulo-spinal, lower limb afferents or cerebellar in origin.

Cranial nerve testing

The most important nerves to test are the facial (CN7) and trigeminal nerves (CN5), as they are affected by lesions in the ear and CPA. CN3, CN4 and CN6 have already been tested in the Section on "Oculomotor Testing", and CN8 with tuning forks, and CN9 and CN10 really require endoscopy. CN11 and CN12 can be easily tested if there is any suspicion of lower brainstem or jugular bulb pathology e.g. with a lateral brainstem lesion.

To test CN7, ask the patient to blink rapidly, this is a more sensitive test than testing the power of eye closure. Even a subtle loss will cause detectable delayed blink in one eyelid compared to the other. This will also test for synkinesis, watch the angle of the mouth for this during blinking. Also test power by trying to forcibly open eyes closed 'as tightly as you can'. Ask the patient to smile and check for symmetry.

Lesions in the brainstem, CPA, temporal bone or parotid can cause CN7 damage.

CN5 is tested with both light touch (ideally with a wisp of cotton, but often with fingers) for symmetry of sensation in upper, middle and lower parts of the face. Technically, this should also be tested with pinprick.

Gross asymmetry of sensation is abnormal. The corneal reflex can also be tested if this is suspected. Lesions of the CPA or trigeminal nerve itself can cause these asymmetries.

Cerebellar testing

Cerebellar lesions can be quite advanced without causing cerebellar findings. It is difficult to test all parts of the cerebellum, as different parts (working together) control posture, oculomotor function, upper limb and lower limb movements. In practice, the oculomotor exam has already been tested, as has posture through gait testing. The lateral parts of the cerebellum are usually tested by two main tests.

The first is 'finger-nose' testing, in which the patient is asked to rapidly and accurately touch their nose, and then your finger, as you keep moving the finger to different fixed positions relative to the patient's nose. Look for coarse intention tremor in the patient's finger trajectory during the finger and nose seeking, inaccuracy in hitting the target, and past-pointing with their finger overshooting your target finger.

Another test is the **dysdiadochokinesia test**, in which the patient is asked to rapidly alternate their hand from prone to supine on the back of their other hand. Cerebellar lesions result in this action looking clumsy and slow. If lower limbs are tested, the patient can be asked to rub one foot smoothly from shin to heel on the other leg, and do it repeatedly, similar to the rapid alternating movements used in all the other cerebellar tests.

Special tests that depend on the history

All the previously mentioned tests are useful to consider in all dizzy patients, as they will exclude serious central pathology. The following tests are usually reserved for patients whose history points towards a specific diagnosis.

Dix–Hallpike positioning

Primarily indicate BPPV. In this test, there is a dynamic and a static component. The aim is to put the posterior semicircular canal in the vertical gravity vector.

The patient is asked again if they have neck stiffness or neck problems before commencing. They are instructed to sit on the stretcher until their head can hang over the edge when they are reclined to lying. Importantly, they are instructed to hold their eyes open even if they are dizzy. The head is grasped firmly from the front or back and brought backwards from the sitting position to lying with the head hanging over the edge of the bed until it is turned 45° towards the test ear, and slightly (about 15°) hanging over the stretcher. The patient eyelids can be held open by the examiner's hand (to avoid eye closure when they get dizzy), and the head held there for at least 45 seconds before it is considered a negative test (Figure 4.5).

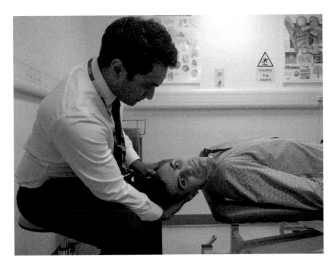

Figure 4.5   When performing the Dix–Hallpike manoeuvre, aim to position the head such that the posterior semicircular canal is in line with gravity.

The typical nystagmus for PC-BPPV is torsional with the fast rotational component beating towards the ground (geotropic), and can have a slight upbeat component (depending on eye-in-head position). The typical nystagmus has all the following features: A latency of about 5–20 seconds, torsional geotropic, a crescendo–decrescendo phase, lasts less than 1 minute, and reverses direction on sitting up (although a particle repositioning manoeuvre may be done instead of sitting the patient up). It must also be associated with subjective vertigo.

Another rarer type of nystagmus for BPPV is the horizontal direction-changing nystagmus, either towards the dependant ear (geotrophic horizontal nystagmus) or away from the dependant ear (ageotropic horizontal nystagmus). Note, the direction depends on which ear is down, even though it arises from the lateral canal of one ear.

Positional downbeat nystagmus can also occur, and can be central, or most often is idiopathic.

Fistula testing

This is a test for a 'third window' such as a superior canal dehiscence or a lateral canal fistula (e.g. from cholesteatoma).

The external ear canal is pressurised with a finger or a Siegel pneumatic speculum, and the eyes are watched carefully under Frenzel's lenses.

> With superior canal dehiscence, nystagmus is not usually seen, but rather a single torsional vertical movement is seen away from the pressurised ear and upwards. This can be very subtle. With a lateral canal fistula, findings depend on where the fistula is and the disease, but most often a slow phase away from the ear is seen with fast phase towards the ear or frank nystagmus beating towards the ear.

Oscillopsia testing

This should be performed if bilateral vestibular loss is suspected, in which the VOR is not available to stabilise the visual image on the retina with concurrent head movements. These patients will also have poor balance on gait testing.

The patient is asked (with their visual aids on if needed) to read the lowest (smallest letters) line they can on a Snellen chart, ideally from 6 feet away if it is a 6 ft chart. The head is then rapidly perturbed in all directions (i.e. up and down and side to side) in small movements in an unpredictable manner so that the patient cannot use smooth pursuit (too rapid) or predictive saccades (too unpredictable) and the patient is asked to read down to the lowest level they can while this is being done.

If the patient drops more than three lines on the chart, this is considered abnormal.

Tests of lateral brainstem dysfunction

These can be useful in the acute emergent setting with acute vertigo. Tests of skew deviation are performed by asking the patient to look at a target covering and uncovering one eye. If there is a skew deviation, when the eye is covered it will move vertically away from the target, and when uncovered it will re-fixate by moving vertically back onto the target.

A Horner's syndrome (ptosis, pupillary constriction [meiosis] and enopthalmos) can also be a sign of lateral brainstem lesion. Other signs are CN dysfunction and cerebellar signs on the lesion side.

Hyperventilation

Forced hyperventilation for 1 minute can be a useful test in chronic dizziness and can reproduce the symptoms of dizziness. It can also unmask retrocochlear pathology by causing nystagmus to the side of the lesion (typically with a vestibular schwannoma) or away from the lesion in severe unilateral vestibular loss.

Otoscopy and tuning fork tests

These tests should not be forgotten in the dizziness exam. Tuning fork tests can demonstrate a distortion and recruitment in the affected ear in Meniere disease, a conductive hearing loss if cholesteatoma is suspected as a cause of a fistula and can refer to the affected side in superior canal dehiscence (and can be heard on the ankle [128 Hz] in this case). They can also be used to test for dorsal column function (using 128 Hz forks) if ascending neuropathy or spinal lesions are suspected as causes of balance loss. Toe joint position testing can confirm this.

Overall advice

Look for patterns that fit together for example if there is bilateral vestibular loss, then gait, head-thrust and oscillopsia testing should all be abnormal. If there is superior canal dehiscence, then the Weber's should lateralise, the tuning fork should be heard on the ankle, there may be a positive fistula test. If there is a unilateral vestibular loss then there should be a positive head thrust, post head-shake nystagmus, possible post-hyperventilation nystagmus (depending on cause if retrocochlear) and mild imbalance on Unterberger's if compensated.

COMMON HEAD AND NECK VIVA TOPICS

EDITED BY JAMES O'HARA

5

- Benign laryngeal lesions
- Deep neck space infections
- Hypercalcaemia and hypocalcaemia
- Hypopharyngeal cancer
- Laryngeal cancer
- Nasopharyngeal cancer
- Neck dissection and accessory nerve palsy
- Obstructive sleep apnoea
- Oral cavity cancer
- Oropharyngeal cancer
- Penetrating neck trauma
- Pharyngeal pouch
- Post-laryngectomy care
- Post-laryngectomy complications
- Radiotherapy, chemotherapy and osteoradionecrosis
- Ranula
- Salivary gland malignancy
- Sialolithiasis
- Thyroid pathology
- Unknown primary cancer in the head and neck
- Vocal cord palsy

Benign Laryngeal Lesions

CHADWAN AL-YAGHCHI

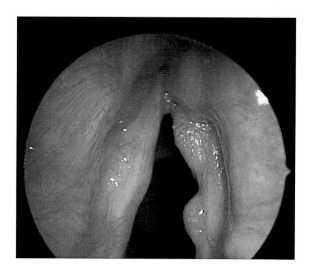

You examine the larynx of a 38-year-old man. Can you describe the clinical findings?

'This is an endoscopic image of the larynx showing multiple papillomatous lesions involving the full length of the right vocal cord and extending to the anterior commissure. There is a similar lesion involving the right false cord anteriorly. These are likely to be papilloma and if recurrent these findings are in keeping with recurrent respiratory papillomatosis (RRP)'.

Important elements in the history

- Voice change, airway compromise including onset, duration and progression
- Smoking and alcohol history
- History of oropharyngeal papilloma
- Immunosuppression

How do you manage this patient?

The likely diagnosis and natural history of the disease should be explained to the patient.

The patient should be offered either a microlaryngoscopy under GA or a period of observation followed by reassessment. Endoscopic examination should include the subglottis and trachea down to the carina with biopsies as required. Tracheal papillomatosis has a higher risk of malignant transformation.

Disease can be debulked using cold steel, microdebrider, KTP (potassium-titanyl-phosphate) or CO_2 laser.

In expert hands all these methods have comparable outcomes. Describe the techniques you have used in the past. If you don't have personal experience, then suggest the use of a microdebrider using a skimmer (least aggressive) blade. Be prepared to explain with drawings where you would make any laser incisions.

Know the five layers of the adult vocal cord – epithelium, lamina propria (superficial, intermediate, deep layers) and vocalis muscle. The vocal ligament is composed of the intermediate and deep layers of the lamina propria.

If the anterior commissure is involved then a staged procedure should be considered to reduce the risk of anterior web formation.

What is the aetiology? Is there risk of malignant transformation?

RRP is caused by human papillomavirus (HPV). Most common serotypes are 6 and 11. The latter is associated with more aggressive disease.

The risk of malignant transformation in laryngeal RRP is low. The risk is much higher if the disease spreads to the trachea. Biopsies should be taken during every procedure and if it shows signs of dysplasia then it should be treated accordingly, with transoral laser resection or radiotherapy as options, followed by close clinical monitoring.

Are you aware of any other treatments?

There are various adjuvant medical treatments in use. The evidence of efficacy is limited to case series. These include:

- Quadrivalent HPV vaccine
- Intralesional cidofovir injection at the time of surgical debulking with repeat every 4–6 weeks
- Bevacizumab (Avastin®) either systemic or intralesional

Other Benign Laryngeal Lesions

Can you describe the clinical findings in this image?

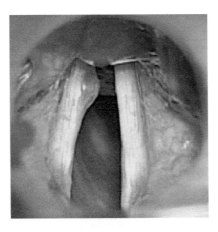

'This is an endoscopic image of the larynx showing a lesion of the anterior left vocal cord. The appearance is in keeping with a vocal cord cyst. There are no overt signs of dysplasia or malignancy'.

Investigations should include videostroboscopy examination and review in a joint voice clinic alongside a speech and language therapist. Given the benign appearance of this lesion microlaryngoscopy is not indicated. Treatment is conservative or surgical with cold steel excision preserving the mucosa of the vibrating edge of the vocal fold. Post-operatively voice rest for 3 days is often recommended with early voice therapy ideally within 2 weeks.

Vocal cord polyps (shown in image below): This could be inflammatory or haemorrhagic. Treatment options are similar to vocal fold cysts. Other options include steroid injection or KTP laser to the feeding blood vessel. Vocal cord polyps can recur and follow up is advised.

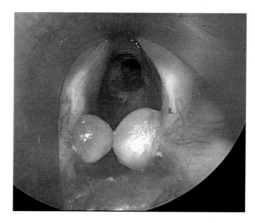

Vocal cord granuloma (contact granuloma): This is a benign lesion arising over the vocal process of the arytenoid cartilage (posterior third of the vocal cord). Commonly they are unilateral and idiopathic but they can occur after intubation. Anti-reflux therapy should be considered including alginates, PPIs and lifestyle modifications. In patients who do not benefit from medical treatment surgical excision may be considered. The latter can be combined with steroid injection to reduce the risk of recurrence. Other options for the management of persistent or recurrent granuloma include botulinum toxin injection to the vocal cord on the ipsilateral side to reduce friction.

Vocal cord nodules: These are most common in professional voice users i.e. singers and teachers. Voice therapy is the main stay of treatment. Vocal coaching and singing lessons are useful to address bad vocal habits. Persistent nodules may be excised.

Reinke's oedema (shown in image below): More common in female smokers. First line of treatment is conservative with smoking cessation. Surgical options include microlaryngoscopy and biopsy to exclude malignancy, lateral cordotomy and aspiration, and KTP laser.

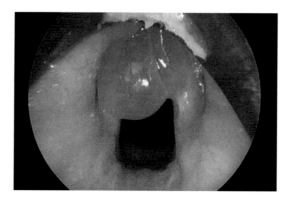

Deep Neck Space Infections

MOHIEMEN ANWAR

Please describe the image

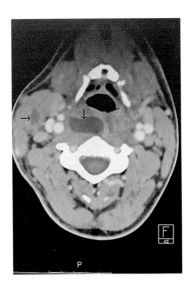

'*This is an axial CT with contrast of the neck at the level of the larynx with evidence of a parapharyngeal and retropharyngeal collection suggestive of an abscess. There is also evidence of oedema of the right sternocleidomastoid (SCM) and another small collection within the muscle*'.

Parapharyngeal abscess is a surgical emergency that needs immediate attention and treatment. In the examination, at least one emergency viva topic will be discussed, and parapharyngeal abscess is a common ENT emergency.

What is your differential diagnosis?

 • Parapharyngeal abscess
 • Retropharyngeal abscess
 • Haematoma
 • Neoplasia

What is a parapharyngeal abscess?

'*A parapharyngeal abscess is a deep neck space infection, inflammation and collection of pus within the parapharyngeal space in the neck*'.

The parapharyngeal space is an inverted pyramid with a base at the skull base and apex at the hyoid. Boundaries are as follows:

- *Superiorly*: Skull base and foramen lacerum
- *Inferiorly*: Greater cornu of the hyoid
- *Medially*: Pretracheal layer of the deep cervical fascia
- *Laterally*: Mandible, lateral pterygoid muscle and parotid gland
- *Anteriorly*: Medial pterygoid muscle and pterygomandibular raphe
- *Posteriorly*: Prevertebral fascia

The parapharyngeal space connects to the retropharyngeal space (abscess formation in this space is common in childhood, due to the involvement of the retropharyngeal lymph nodes). The retropharyngeal space extends to the superior mediastinum at the level of T2 vertebrae, hence when suspected imaging should include the chest. The parapharyngeal space also connects to the submandibular space via the pterygomandibular raphe.

Parapharyngeal abscess are also commonly complications of tonsillitis, dental infections and supraglottitis. It can also originate from skin and sinus infections.

How would you manage a patient with a parapharyngeal abscess?

Assess if the patient is stable first.

- Use the ABC approach
- Secure airway if the airway is compromised
- Manage in resus with a full resuscitation team including anaesthetist

If the airway is stable:

History:

- Worsening history of sore throat, dysphagia and odynophagia
- Fitness for GA, last meal, allergies

Examination:

- ABC
- Hot potato voice and trismus due to the involvement of pterygoid muscles
- Torticollis
- Systemically unwell, septic, pyrexial
- Drooling and stertor

- Neck swelling
- Neck palpation for swelling and lymphadenopathy
- Neck movements
- Oral cavity for tonsillitis/quinsy
- Flexible nasendoscopy: Parapharyngeal swelling and asymmetry, any airway compromise

Investigation:

- Bloods: FBC, U+E, CRP, blood cultures
- CT neck (+ chest) with contrast
- USS neck and potential guided aspiration (if appropriate e.g. small, accessible collection)

Treatment:

- Broad spectrum IV antibiotics (each trust has their own microbiology guidelines which should be accessed. Co-amoxiclav or cefuroxime and metronidazole are common options. The risk of *Clostridium difficile* should be appreciated and means to reduce this risk e.g. changing PPI to H2 antagonists, reducing to an oral dose when clinical improvement occurs).
- Manage in ITU/HDU setup with regular close monitoring
- If CT shows small abscess and undetermined inflammatory reaction but no frank abscess then:
  - Discuss with microbiology
  - Continue IV Abx with close clinical and WCC/CRP monitoring
  - Be prepared to repeat CT if no clinical improvement or deterioration in 24–48 hours
- If CT shows a 'significant' abscess formation (>2.5 cm)
  - Surgery: Transcervical approach

    Transverse skin crease incision or incision along the anterior border of SCM. The latter affords improved access to the clivus and root of neck but gives an inferior cosmetic scar); identify the gutter between the SCM and strap muscles. Control the middle thyroid vein. The common facial vein can be ligated for improved access. Bluntly dissect (using an artery forceps or finger dissection) towards the skull base/clivus superiorly and to the root of the neck inferiorly. Dissection of loculi that meet the retropharyngeal space and beyond to join the contralateral parapharyngeal space should be performed. Irrigate and leave a corrugated drain which should be inserted to the limits of the abscess cavity both superiorly and inferiorly.
  - For severe abscesses with airway compromise, or those with a prolonged period of intubation predicted (e.g. Ludwig's angina or bilateral parapharyngeal abscess) consider a tracheostomy.
  - Surgery: Transoral approach in small accessible abscess by deroofing the abscess

Inform the anaesthetist of the risk of deroofing the collection during intubation and the risk of aspiration. Fibreoptic intubation might be the preferred option of intubation in this situation.

Consider inserting an NG tube for feeding to improve healing. Consider a water-soluble swallowing assessment in 72 hours post-operatively.

Consider repeating the scan if no clinical improvement or deterioration.

If left undrained, what are the risks associated with deep neck space infections?

- Mediastinitis
- Airway compromise
- Infection of neck planes and perforation of viscus
- Fistula formation
- IJV thrombosis and necrosis of carotid
- Skull base infection and CN involvement
- Chest infection and pericardial infections

Hypercalcaemia and Hypocalcaemia

ZI-WEI LIU

Whilst this has not been a common examination topic, it is not inconceivable that you could be asked about either of these scenarios.

What is primary hyperparathyroidism?

'*Primary hyperparathyroidism is caused by excess secretion of PTH. In 80% of cases this is due to a single parathyroid adenoma, and in 20% of cases multi-gland hyperplasia is the cause*'.

How would you select patients for surgery?

Most patients are asymptomatic. The Fourth International Workshop on asymptomatic primary hyperparathyroidism has set out guidelines for management. Patients meeting one of the following should be considered for surgical intervention:

- Serum calcium of 0.25 mmol/L above normal
- Bone density more than 2.5 sd below peak bone mass (T-score <2.5)
- Previous asymptomatic vertebral fracture
- eGFR <60 mL/min
- 24 hour urinary calcium >10 mmol/day
- Renal stones
- Age less than 50 years

Bilezikian JP. Guidelines for the management of asymptomatic primary hyperparathyroidism: Summary statement from the fourth international workshop. *J Clin Endocrinol Metab.* 2014;99:3561–9.

Symptomatic patients (e.g. renal stones, fractures) should have parathyroid surgery.

What investigations would you choose to localise parathyroid adenomas pre-op?

Sestamibi, SPECT, US and MRI have all been used to localise parathyroid adenomas pre-op.

There is no single best modality so most centres will use a combination of two modalities to confirm location. 99mTc-sestamibi with neck USS will accurately locate parathyroid adenomas in 79%–95% of cases. Four-dimensional CT probably has the highest sensitivity but radiation dose is >50 times higher than a sestamibi scan.

Bilateral four-gland exploration should be considered where imaging results are discordant, or where previous selective parathyroidectomy has failed. Intraoperative PTH levels and frozen sections can be used to ensure the adenoma has been removed.

What signs and symptoms would you find in a patient with hypocalcaemia?

The commonest scenario presenting to ENT surgeons is the patient with acute hypocalcaemia following total thyroidectomy. Symptoms typically manifest when corrected calcium levels fall below 1.9 mmol/L. These include peri-oral tingling, Trousseau's sign, Chvostek's sign, tetany, laryngospasm, prolonged QT interval and seizures.

How would you investigate a patient with hypocalcaemia post thyroidectomy?

Investigations should include serum calcium, PTH (normal PTH usually predicts quick recovery), urea and electrolytes, phosphate and magnesium. An ECG should be performed.

How do you manage a patient with acute hypocalcaemia post thyroidectomy?

The Society for Endocrinology's Emergency Management of Acute Hypocalcaemia guidelines (2016) suggest:

- Mild hypocalcaemia (serum calcium 1.9–2.1 mmol/L), oral calcium supplements BD. Start alfacalcidol if hypocalcaemia persists beyond 72 hrs on oral calcium
- Severe hypocalcaemia: Serum calcium <1.9 mmol/L or symptomatic at any level below reference range should be treated as a medical emergency. Commence treatment with IV calcium gluconate initially 10–20 mL of 10%, followed by a 100 mL 10% calcium gluconate diluted in 1 L of normal saline infusion. Cardiac monitoring is required and endocrine advice should be sought.

Hypopharyngeal Cancer

LAURA WARNER

Please describe this image

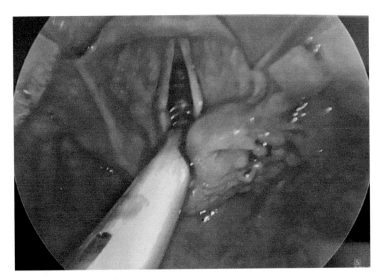

'This is an endoscopic picture of the larynx and hypopharynx of an intubated patient. There is an irregular lesion of the right hypopharynx, involving the medial wall of the piriform fossa and the aryepiglottic fold that is suspicious for a hypopharyngeal malignancy'.

What are the anatomical subsites of the hypopharynx? Which is most commonly affected by tumours?

The subsites are the piriform fossa, posterior hypopharyngeal wall and the post cricoid area. The majority of cancers are found in the piriform fossa (65%–80%), with 10%–20% in the posterior pharyngeal wall and 5%–15% in the post cricoid area.

Key features in the history:

 • Onset and progression of symptoms: Pain, odynophagia, dysphagia, dysphonia, otalgia
- Weight loss, current nutritional status
- Risk factors: Smoking, alcohol intake
- Past medical history, previous head and neck cancer treatment, estimate performance status
- Family/social support

What are your initial steps in managing this patient?

The key initial steps in managing this patient are to stage the disease by expediently arranging for cross-sectional imaging of the neck and chest (CT or MRI neck, CT thorax) and pharyngoscopy and biopsy.

It is important to also offer the patient analgesia and to request nutritional supplements or arrange for a dietician review if they have reduced oral intake.

> This aspect of care is frequently omitted from viva answers but mentioning this shows that you adopt a holistic and caring approach to managing this patient.

When would you request a PET-CT for a patient with hypopharyngeal SCC?

PET-CT is indicated for primary T4 hypopharyngeal lesions, or for patients with N3 disease. PET-CT is indicated for recurrent hypopharyngeal SCC if radical treatment is being considered.

 Ensure you are familiar with the 2016 NICE (National Institute for Health and Care Excellence) guidelines for the assessment and management of cancer of the upper aerodigestive tract.

What are the treatment options for hypopharyngeal cancer?

> All cases should be discussed at the head and neck MDT but you should be able to talk to the examiner about the treatment options. It is worth practising a succinct sentence to explain that you would discuss at the MDT and involve the entire team in care – the CNS team, SLT, dieticians etc.

Treatment options include primary radiotherapy/chemoradiotherapy or surgery with adjuvant (chemo) radiotherapy. Treatment decisions are based on the tumour stage, the patient's symptoms and performance status and patient preference for example if the patient has a compromised airway or swallow pre-treatment they may be better treated with surgery, as (chemo)radiotherapy will not improve function and may worsen the situation.

Transoral resection (laser or robotic) is possible for small, accessible lesions, however the mainstay of surgical treatment of hypopharyngeal SCC is total laryngectomy, partial pharyngectomy and may require reconstruction.

 Read about the flaps that are commonly used for pharyngeal reconstruction i.e. pedicled flap (pectoralis major) and free flaps (radial forearm or antero-lateral thigh [ALT] flap).

Non-surgical treatment with radical radiotherapy or concurrent chemoradiotherapy offers organ preservation but carries a risk of short- and long-term side effects. Meta-analysis data from the MACH-NC study demonstrates that addition of chemotherapy to radiotherapy improves 5-year survival for HNSCC by 4% in patients under 71 but significantly increases toxicity. There is no survival benefit in patients over 71.

Pignon JP, Bourhis J, Domenge C et al. Chemotherapy added to locoregional treatment for HNSCC: Three meta-analyses of updated individual data. MACH-NC Collaborative Group. Meta-Analysis of CT on Head and Neck Cancer; *Lancet.* 2000;355(9208):949–55.

What is the prognosis for hypopharyngeal cancer?

The overall 5-year survival for all stages of hypopharyngeal cancer is 30% (compared to 65% for oropharyngeal cancer). For T1/T2 lesions it is 60%.

Why is the prognosis of hypopharyngeal cancer poor?

The key reasons why the prognosis is poor are:

- Later presentation: 80% are stage III at presentation
- High propensity for bilateral, multi-level nodal metastasis. Extra-nodal extension is common
- Early distant metastasis: Highest rates of distant metastasis for all HNSCC

Laryngeal Cancer

LAURA WARNER

Please describe this image

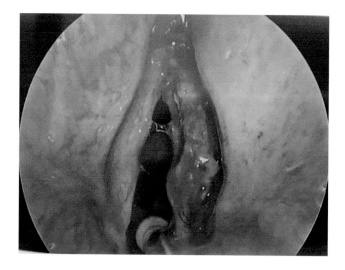

'This is an endoscopic picture of a larynx, in a patient intubated with a jet-ventilation catheter. The right vocal cord is irregular and erythematous lesion with areas of leukoplakia. This is highly suspicious for a laryngeal malignancy'.

Important points to cover in the history

 • Onset and progression of voice change
- Pain, otalgia
- Swallowing difficulties, weight loss
- Risk factors: Smoking, alcohol intake
- Past medical history, previous head and neck cancer treatment, estimate performance status
- Occupation and hobbies relevant to voice use
- Family/social support

What imaging would you request for this patient?

Investigation of head and neck cancer depends on the suspected clinical stage as T1/T2 N0 tumours do not require full **systemic** staging, according to the 2016 NICE guidelines.

Neck staging is not indicated where the risk of occult nodal disease is less than 15% and many early laryngeal cancers are too small to be detected by imaging. If there are suspected adverse features such as cartilage invasion from anterior commissure involvement imaging is indicated as it may provide vital information for treatment planning. If you think this is the case tell the examiners why you would order a scan, be prepared to defend your answer.

Don't forget to say you would order a CXR to rule out synchronous lung primary, however many institutions still advocate CT thorax as the incidence of synchronous lung primary cancers is reported at between 5% and 19%.

 Ensure you are familiar with the 2016 NICE guidelines for the assessment and management of cancer of the upper aerodigestive tract.

Talk me through the T-staging of laryngeal cancer. How would you stage this lesion?

It is important to be familiar with the TNM classification for head and neck cancers. Be succinct in your answer and give the defining features of each stage.

The image shown appears to be T1a as it is confined to one vocal cord. You would need to know about cord mobility and invasion of other subsites (i.e. subglottis and ventricle – which you cannot tell from this picture) so you can either ask the examiner or say:

'*Assuming the cord is mobile and does not invade other subsites it is a T1a lesion. As part of the microlaryngoscopy or endoscopic examination, I would pay particular attention to the anterior commissure, subglottis and ventricle. Angled Hopkins rods are particularly useful in this respect*'.

What treatment options do you know about for early laryngeal cancer and what would you suggest for this patient?

All cases should be discussed at the head and neck MDT. Transoral surgery and radiotherapy are both appropriate treatment options for this patient, with both offering 5-year local control with survival over 95%. Open partial laryngectomy may be indicated for some T2 lesions if transoral surgery is not feasible.

'*For this patient with T1a glottic SCC I would advocate transoral laser surgery as it is a single, convenient treatment, which avoids the potential side effects of radiotherapy and keeps radiotherapy as an option for recurrence. NICE guidelines now recommend offering transoral laser microsurgery for T1a tumours. Some clinicians feel that radiotherapy may offer better voice outcomes for some T1a tumours. Voice outcomes should be discussed with the patient to aid decision making*'.

	Transoral laser surgery	Radiotherapy
Advantages	Single, day case treatment Can be repeated to ensure clearance Cost advantage Preserves radiotherapy as salvage option	Improved voice outcomes (in some areas i.e. anterior commissure) No anaesthetic required
Disadvantages	Potentially poorer voice outcomes May not be possible if access difficult	Course of treatment Long-term swallowing dysfunction May prohibit transoral laser microsurgery if recurrence

Be ready to discuss the evidence to support your choice.

O'Hara J, Markey A, Homer J. Transoral laser surgery versus radiotherapy for tumour stage 1a or 1b glottic squamous cell carcinoma: Systematic review of local control outcomes; *J Laryngol Otol.* 2013;127(8):732–8.

Warner L, Lee K, Homer J. Transoral laser microsurgery versus radiotherapy for T2 glottic squamous cell carcinoma: A systematic review of local control outcomes; *Clin Otolaryngol.* 2017;42(3):629–36.

Do you know a classification system for laser laryngeal surgery?

European Laryngological society classification of transoral laser cordectomy:

- *Type I:* Subepithelial cordectomy
- *Type II*: Subligamental cordectomy
- *Type III*: Transmuscular cordectomy
- *Type IV*: Total cordectomy
- *Type V*: Extended cordectomy:
  - *Va*: Involving the contralateral vocal cord
  - *Vb*: Involving the ipsilateral arytenoid
  - *Vc*: Involving the laryngeal ventricle
  - *Vd*: Involving subglottis
- *Type VI*: Cordectomy for anterior commissure carcinoma

Remacle M, Van Haverbeke C, Exckel H et al. Proposal for revision of the European Laryngological Society classification of endoscopic cordectomies; *Eur Arch Oto-Rhino-Laryngol.* 2007;264(5);499–504.

What are the options for treating locally advanced laryngeal cancer (T3/T4)? How would you choose between these options?

The choice here is between surgery (total laryngectomy and neck dissections) with adjuvant radiotherapy (±chemotherapy) or organ preservation treatment with radiotherapy or concurrent chemoradiotherapy. This should follow a shared decision-making process with active involvement of patients and their families. National guidelines state that most patients with T3 and T4 tumours, which do not invade through the thyroid cartilage into soft tissue, are suitable for organ preservation non-surgical treatment.

In patients with pre-treatment airway or swallowing impairment organ preservation strategies may result in inadequate laryngeal function after treatment and many of these patients will require long-term enteral feeding and/or tracheostomy. Because of this, patients may opt for total laryngectomy if their breathing or swallowing are significantly affected before treatment. Patients with cartilage invasion or extra-laryngeal spread are unlikely to be cured with (chemo) radiotherapy and should be offered primary surgery.

Where expertise exists, some T3 tumours may be suitable for open partial laryngeal surgery.

 Forastiere A, Goepfert H, Maor M et al. Concurrent chemotherapy and radiotherapy for organ preservation in advanced laryngeal cancer; *N Engl J Med.* 2003;349(22):2091–8.

Nasopharyngeal Cancer

JASON FLEMING

Please describe this image

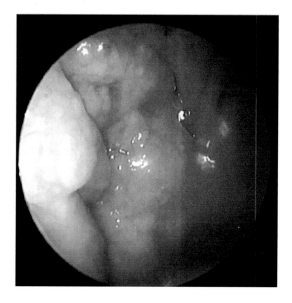

'*This is a clinical endoscopic photograph of a post-nasal space. The most obvious abnormality is a mass filling the right fossa of Rosenmuller and adjacent nasopharynx which appears to extend to the midline, but the inferior extent is not fully seen. The appearance is consistent with a NPC*'.

What would be the important aspects in the history?

Do not waste valuable time giving a long and irrelevant list of a generic patient history. Examiners are looking for salient points specifically relevant to NPC. Imagine you are presenting in the head and neck MDT and mention those points that the team members present would want to know:

- Age
- Ethnicity (highly prevalent in Southern China and North Africa)
- EBV history
- Family history
- Nasal and aural symptoms
- CN nerve symptoms
- Neck lumps
- PMH (past medical history) and performance status

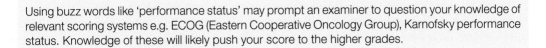

Using buzz words like 'performance status' may prompt an examiner to question your knowledge of relevant scoring systems e.g. ECOG (Eastern Cooperative Oncology Group), Karnofsky performance status. Knowledge of these will likely push your score to the higher grades.

How would you investigate this patient?

'*Clinical evaluation with flexible and/or rigid nasendoscopy should be followed by imaging investigations to ideally complete staging before proceeding to biopsies in theatre. Staging investigations should include CT imaging of the head, neck and chest and/or MRI. In my experience PET-CT is being more frequently used for patients with advanced stage disease (T3, T4). As well as pathological examination of biopsies, analysis for EBV-encoded small non-coding RNAs (EBERs) are now commonly performed*'.

Be careful here. Current UK guidelines recommend CT for staging and MRI in cases of advanced disease for more accurate skull base assessment. If you get pressed on imaging then you can emphasise this but bringing in the option of PET-CT imaging shows that you have experience of managing this condition and are aware of the concern regarding distant metastases in this disease.

Do you know any classification systems for NPC?

This is a good opportunity to show your knowledge. Discuss use of the WHO pathological classification dividing disease into keratinising (formerly type I) and the more prevalent virally-driven nonkeratinizing type, which can be subdivided into differentiated (formerly type II) and undifferentiated (formerly type III) disease. There is also a rare basaloid SCC subtype.

How would you stage this disease?

Once you have demonstrated knowledge of the disease, pathology and diagnostic pathway, you have met the safe practice standard and have now reached the advanced point scoring section of the viva. Changes of AJCC/UICC TNM staging from 7th to 8th edition can complicate this answer but be prepared to list current staging definitions if prompted. However if asked an open question like this one, under exam and limited time pressure, broad statements to demonstrate your understanding, rather than listing every single TNM category, will likely produce a sound and succinct structured answer. An example answer is as follows:

'*Staging is performed using the AJCC/UICC TNM system. The 7th edition specified early stage primary disease as confined locally or with parapharyngeal extension, and later stages involving bony invasion or intracranial/CN extension. The N staging for NPC also differed to other HNSCC by broadly classifying nodes as unilateral, bilateral or large nodes (>6 cm) involving the supraclavicular fossa. Changes in the new 8th edition include downgrading adjacent muscle involvement (pterygoids, prevertebral) from T4 to T2 and combining N3a and b staging into a single N3 category incorporating either size >6 cm or location below the cricoid cartilage*'.

The same patient has had the diagnosis of NPC confirmed and it appears to be early-stage disease. Tell me what treatment options are available.

If you have not had the opportunity yet to say you would discuss treatment options in an MDT setting with oncology teams, now is your chance! Before time runs out it is important to state '*The primary treatment modality for NPC is radiotherapy*'.

If there is further time available to develop your answer you can explain that this is because the location of the disease makes surgical resection difficult and the disease is radiosensitive. IMRT allows better targeted treatment with the benefit of minimising the dose received by normal adjacent tissue. Concurrent chemoradiotherapy with cisplatin-based treatment offers significant improvement in overall survival (6%) in patients with advanced (stage III and IV) disease. The role of adjuvant and induction chemotherapy regimens is less clear and is the subject of ongoing trials.

Again, say what you have seen in your training.

Is there any role for surgery in NPC treatment?

'*In my experience surgery is generally limited to diagnostic procedures. However there is a potential role for salvage surgery at the primary site in the form of nasopharyngectomy (endoscopic or open) due to the high toxicity of re-irradiation. Surgery is more favourable if there is evidence of low disease volume and good patient performance status. Similarly salvage neck dissection is often the treatment of choice for persistent or recurrent disease in the neck, although the high prevalence of ECS often necessitates a radical procedure*'.

 Simo R, Robinson M, Lei M et al. Read nasopharyngeal carcinoma: United Kingdom National Multidisciplinary Guidelines; *J Laryngol Otol*. 2016;130(Suppl 2):S97–S103.

Neck Dissection and Accessory Nerve Palsy

JAGDEEP VIRK

In any of the head and neck vivas you need to be able to interpret operative pictures as well as radiological images.

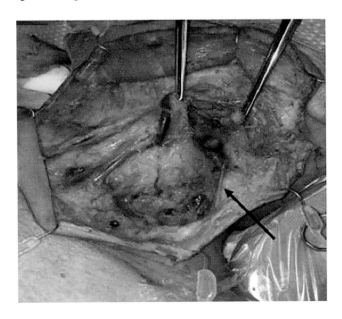

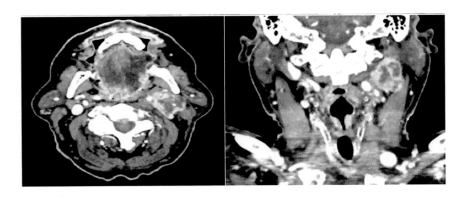

Describe these images. What does the black arrow in the top picture indicate?

'*The lower two images are axial and coronal CT slices, with contrast, demonstrating a likely pathological left level II/III lymph node encasing the region of the carotid bifurcation and reaching the skull base; there are some areas of calcification and possible extracapsular extension. I also note irregularity of the left dorsolateral tongue, which may represent the primary site. The intraoperative image is consistent with a modified radical neck dissection (MRND). The arrow is on the accessory nerve'.*

How would you classify neck dissections?

'A neck dissection is the surgical removal of lymph nodes from the neck'.

The American Head and Neck Society and American Academy of Otolaryngology Head and Neck Surgery (AAOHNS, 2001) classify neck dissection as:

  Radical neck dissection (RND): Removal of all ipsilateral cervical nodes from levels I to V together with the IJV, SCM and SAN.

  MRND: Removal of the same nodes as an RND but with preservation of one or more of the non-lymphatic structures (IJV, SCM, SAN).

  Selective neck dissection (SND): Preservation of one or more of the nodal levels as removed routinely at RND e.g. SND I–III (indicates the removal of ipsilateral levels I, II and III).

  Extended: Removal of nodal levels or non-lymphatic structures not routinely removed at RND e.g. hypoglossal nerve, vagus nerve, skin, digastric muscle.

Neck dissections can also be more broadly considered as elective (i.e. clinicoradiologically N0) and therapeutic (N+).

> For this topic, you must be able to define the levels of the neck and describe the basic incisions/ steps of the procedure.

Can you tell me about skin incisions used for neck dissection?

The incision used will depend on the site of the primary tumour and whether a unilateral or bilateral neck dissection is to be undertaken. The incision must allow adequate exposure of the surgical field whilst maintaining vascularised skin flaps. Other concerns include previous surgical scars, maintaining cosmesis (e.g. by using relaxed skin tension lines) and a consideration of any reconstruction required.

Commonly used incisions are MacFee and Gluck (or apron) incisions. Conley, Schobinger, single or double Y incisions and hockey stick incisions are also used. However, if used, care must be taken with these latter incisions as they may become devascularised.

Rationale for neck dissection

Elective neck dissection is undertaken when the risk of occult neck disease is significant (>15%–20% risk is often quoted). The levels of nodes removed in elective selective neck dissection will be dependent on primary site (e.g. oral cavity level I–III, oropharynx/larynx II–IV).

Therapeutic neck dissection in N+ or salvage setting: The aim is to perform an oncologically sound procedure that preserves non-lymphatic structures where possible (improved functional outcomes).

In some cases, this will not be achievable, as in this case (an MRND or RND will be needed).

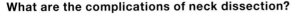

What are the complications of neck dissection?

Always answer this systematically (e.g. early/intermediate/late; local/general).

- *Early:*
  - Local: Bleeding, airway obstruction, increased ICP, carotid sinus syndrome, nerve injury (marginal mandibular, accessory, hypoglossal, vagus, phrenic nerves and brachial plexus), vascular injury leading to stroke.
  - General: Pneumothorax
- *Intermediate:*
  - Local: Seroma, chyle leak, infection, wound dehiscence, carotid artery rupture, fistula
  - General: Bronchopneumonia, basal collapse, DVT
- *Late:* Hypertrophic or keloid scarring, shoulder dysfunction

What are your landmarks to identify the accessory nerve?

- Tendinous part of SCM
- Overlying perforator vessel
- Transverse process of C1
- Erb's point (the nerve lies approximately 1 cm above)
- Usually crosses IJV anteriorly (but can be posterior in about 19% of cases or even run through bifid IJV)
- Deep to posterior belly of digastric

Higher level questions may appear towards the end of the viva. For example:

Do you think level IIb should be dissected in laryngeal and supraglottic cancers? When would you dissect level IIb? What can dissecting there increase the risk of?

Level IIb are nodes postero-lateral to the vertical plane of the accessory nerve.

Dissection increases the risk of skeletonising and devascularising the accessory nerve with resultant shoulder dysfunction requiring early and intensive physiotherapy.

Kou Y, Zhao T, Huang S et al. Cervical level IIb metastases in squamous cell carcinoma of the oral cavity: A systematic review and meta-analysis. *Onco Targets Ther.* 2017;10:4475–83.

Paleri V, Kumar Subramaniam S, Oozeer N et al. Dissection of the submuscular recess in squamous cell cancer of the upper aerodigestive tract. *Head Neck.* 2008;30:194–200.

Here are some of the issues you need to be aware of in regard of dissecting level IIb:

In elective neck dissections, level IIb can be spared. The exception is for parotid malignancies; if an elective neck dissection is merited, level IIb should be dissected. For therapeutic neck dissections, level IIb should be dissected.

Obstructive Sleep Apnoea (OSA)

ZI-WEI LIU

Although more common in the paediatric ENT section (see the separate paediatric OSA chapter in the paediatric ENT section of this book), this subject has been asked before in the context of adult patients.

How is OSA graded?

OSA is episodes of complete or partial airway obstruction during sleep.

Episodes are termed apnoea (cessation of breathing for >10 seconds) or hypopnoea (reduction of airflow by >50%). In adults, mild OSA is AHI of 5–14 episodes/hour, moderate 15–30, and severe >30 episodes/hour.

What would you ask about in the history of a patient with sleep apnoea?

- Unrefreshing sleep, day time somnolence
- Weight gain
- Reported history of apnoeic episodes during sleep
- Snoring (not always correlated with apnoea)
- Past medical history including cardiovascular risk factors (hypertension, diabetes, obesity)
- Alcohol intake or use of sedative type medications
- Epworth sleepiness score (eight scenarios scored 0–3, 0 = would never doze, 3 = high chance of dozing, max score = 24)

How would you examine this patient with OSA/snoring?

Salient examination findings:

- Retrognathia (role of mandibular advancement device)
- Mouth opening
- Tonsil size
- Friedman and Mallampati grading
- Collar size and BMI (BMI greater than 30 predicts poor surgical outcome)
- Flexible nasendoscopy to assess collapse at the palatal/oropharyngeal level using Muller's manoeuvre

What is a 'sleep study'?

The commonest types of sleep study are cardiopulmonary sleep studies and polysomnography. Overnight pulse oximetry alone is often used in children but not in adults.

Cardiopulmonary sleep studies include readings from nasal cannulae (to detect airflow), pulse oximetry, chest and abdominal bands (to detect efforts of respiration) and sometimes ECG. This is the commonest type of sleep study and can distinguish OSA from central sleep apnoea. The results will give an AHI index and ODI (oxygen desaturation index - $\geq 4\%$ shift from baseline).

Polysomnography will have additional readings from EEG and leg movement monitors. This is requested where parasomnias are suspected and is not usually required to diagnose simple OSA.

How would you manage sleep apnoea in an adult patient?

OSA should be managed in conjunction with respiratory physicians.

 NICE guidelines on the management of sleep apnoea (2008) suggest management as follows:

- Mild OSA: Lifestyle changes including weight loss, exercise, mandibular advancement devices, reduction in alcohol intake. CPAP is only indicated if these treatments have failed and the patient has symptoms that affect quality of life (inability to carry out daily activities).
- Moderate and severe OSA is treated primarily with CPAP.

Surgery is indicated for failure to tolerate CPAP treatment and mild OSA where surgery is the patient's preference. Surgery alone may improve moderate or severe sleep apnoea but is unlikely to be curative in the long term without other modalities of treatment.

What are the surgical options for OSA?

Some advocate an assessment under anaesthesia (drug-induced sleep endoscopy, DISE) which identifies anatomical targets although this is not widely practised in the UK.

Candidates should be aware of recent changes in commissioning guidelines. Some areas of the country are now unable to offer surgical intervention in the NHS. This is due to a lack of high-quality evidence in support of surgical interventions (which is different to evidence showing a lack of effectiveness).

Surgical options include nasal surgery (septoplasty, inferior turbinate reduction, polypectomy; when significant nasal obstruction may be contributing to the sleep disordered breathing) tonsillectomy, uvulopalatoplasty and more rarely tongue base reduction (robotic surgery has been described). Less commonly performed operations include mandibular advancement, hyoid suspension and more recently, implantable hypoglossal nerve stimulators.

How would you advise a patient with OSA on driving?

OSA only needs to be reported to the DVLA if there is excessive sleepiness having, or likely to have, an adverse effect on driving. This should be backed up by a clinical assessment and sleep study. Clinicians should advise patients of the need to notify DVLA if they have moderate to severe sleep apnoea with sleepiness likely to impact driving. There is no obligation on clinicians to check whether the patient is compliant with advice, but if they become aware that patients are driving against advice, they should inform the DVLA (patient consent is not required) and write a letter notifying the patient that this is going to be the case.

 Further guidance: British Thoracic Society position statement on driving and OSA 2018.

Oral Cavity Cancer

JASON FLEMING

Describe this clinical photograph

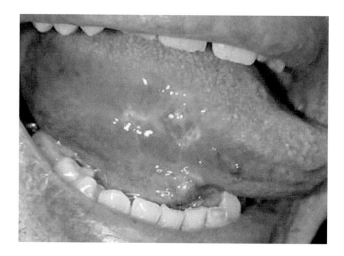

'*The most obvious abnormality is a lesion on the right lateral border of the anterior tongue. The lesion appears indurated with central erythema and ulceration. Whilst this lesion could represent an aphthous, inflammatory or trauma related ulcer, my main concern is an SCC*'.

What are risk factors in the history that would make you more concerned?

- Risk factors: Smoking, alcohol intake. If the patient was a current or recent ex-smoker, his/her risk of oral SCC, by far the most common oral malignancy, triples and a significant alcohol intake acts synergistically to increase the likelihood of this disease over 10-fold
- Past medical history: Previous head and neck cancer treatment
- Ethnic origin: If the patient was of Asian or Indian descent remember to also specifically ask about areca (betel) nut/paan chewing.

How would you investigate and stage this disease?

Clinical assessment and cross-sectional imaging (CT/MRI) is the cornerstone of pre-operative assessment to accurately stage the disease according to AJCC/UICC staging system. Both imaging modalities are useful in certain scenarios and often combined; CT provides excellent information on bony invasion and MRI provides improved soft tissue resolution. CT images of the primary tumour can be affected significantly by dental amalgam.

Many MDTs now have specific guidelines on first-line imaging and in this case, you can state your local guidelines in your answer to demonstrate your experience of your regional MDT. Primary lesions will require a biopsy which, unless the lesion is small, will often involve incisional or mapping biopsies. Ideally these should be performed after imaging as subsequent MRI for example would significantly over estimate the size of the lesion due to post-operative inflammation. Imaging should include both the neck and a CT chest (with contrast) to complete staging.

How do you treat the primary disease?

Surgery is the mainstay of treatment. A primary en-bloc resection with a minimum of 5 mm final pathological margins is the gold standard surgical aim and a pre-operative decision should be made how best to achieve this result. A number of approaches are possible depending on the site and stage of the primary tumour. Transoral excision comprises the most common approach although significant oropharyngeal extension or trismus is the main contraindications to this technique. A visor flap with lingual release allows a drop-down technique, allowing the primary tumour to be excised in continuity with the neck dissection. While this allows a more controlled floor of mouth and posterior tongue excision, repair of the floor of mouth with appropriate reconstructive techniques must then be considered in order to separate the anatomical spaces that have been joined in the resection. Finally, mandibulotomy, usually combined with lip split, allows access to large tumours. Maintenance of occlusion and cosmetic complications due to the lip and skin incisions both need consideration and numerous modifications of technique have been recommended to minimise morbidity. In very advanced disease or patients with significant comorbidities, palliative approaches may be appropriate.

The tumour is suspected to involve the mandibular cortex: How will this change your planned surgery?

Mandibular involvement indicates advanced disease but pre-operative imaging (CT), intraoperative assessment and patient factors ultimately dictate the extent of mandibulectomy required. With disease extending to the cortex or superficial periosteal invasion only, in a dentate patient with adequate vertical mandibular height, a marginal mandibulectomy may suffice. However, this is not always possible and any negative prognostic disease or patient factors may dictate a segmental mandibulectomy with appropriate reconstruction.

When would you perform a neck dissection?

'When the risk of occult neck disease is greater than 20% or for any N+ neck disease'.

The examiners will be wanting a little more detail on the potential options for treatment here but as an opening statement, this is a strong start and demonstrates your knowledge of the overriding rationale behind the surgical approach to the neck in malignant disease.

Key points that you can expand on as required are:

- Overall occult neck disease in all oral cavity SCC is approximately 30%
- Level I evidence demonstrates an improved survival in cN0 patients with elective neck dissection compared with surveillance and therapeutic neck dissection

D'Cruz AK, Vaish R, Kapre N et al. Elective versus therapeutic neck dissection in node-negative oral cancer. *N Engl J Med*. 2015;373(6):521–9.

- Sentinel node biopsy is a new technique in HNSCC for early stage oral tumours to stage the neck and can help determine who requires a formal neck dissection.
- A supraomohyoid (levels I–III) neck dissection is usually sufficient in cN0 patients due to the low incidence of isolated occult level IV disease.
- In a disease-positive neck, a therapeutic selective neck dissection is still usually oncologically sound, although there is more controversy around level IV; a formal level V dissection is rarely required.
- Multiple positive nodes, bulky disease or clinically/radiologically likely extracapsular extension will often require a more extensive resection in the form of a MRND.

As the favoured modality treatment for oral cavity cancer is usually surgery, the same modality is recommended to treat the neck prophylactically (in the N0 neck) or therapeutically (in the N+ neck) at the same operation, unless the disease is minimally invasive. This has the added advantage of facilitating the exposure and access to vessels if free flap reconstruction is required.

'Ultimately, tailoring the extent of neck dissection to the extent of the disease using all available pre- and intraoperative assessment methods is a safe and sound approach'.

Describe what you know about principles of reconstruction in oral surgery

The reconstructive ladder should be considered in this setting to how best restore form and function. The size and site of the defect and patient factors will ultimately determine the reconstructive options, from leaving small oral cavity defects to heal by secondary intention, through to complex osseocutaneous microvascular free flaps following significant mandibular resection. Small partial glossectomy defects can often be closed with primary closure or left to heal by secondary intention. Local flaps in the oral cavity such as the submental island flap are another option for other small defects. Larger tongue defects may require free flap reconstruction to optimise speech and swallowing, such as the radial forearm free flap, through to the ALT flap for larger subtotal or total glossectomy defects. If free flap reconstruction is not appropriate, either due to patient-related factors or service provision, pedicled flaps such as the pectoralis major musculocutaneous flap are a very reasonable option.

What is the role of external beam radiotherapy in treating this disease?

'Due to the side effects of radiotherapy on oral cavity mucosa and the risk of osteoradionecrosis (ORN) at the doses required for radical treatment, this modality is not usually recommended as a primary curative option. Post operative radiotherapy (PORT) however has been shown to improve locoregional control and overall survival in locally advanced cancers. PORT should be considered in all patients with bulky T3 or T4 tumours and N2 disease or above. Other prognostic features such as perineural/lymphovascular invasion should also be discussed in the MDT setting for patients who do not fit the criteria for a patient-tailored approach. Positive margins or ECS are indications for consideration of adjuvant chemoradiotherapy depending on patient factors e.g. age, comorbidities, performance status'.

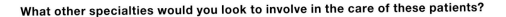

What other specialties would you look to involve in the care of these patients?

Remembering the members of the team who contribute to the MDT should make this question straightforward. Outside of the primary treating ablative and reconstructive surgeons and oncologists, an appreciation of the pre-, peri- and post-op management of these patients should ensure you remember all relevant teams which may include cancer nurse specialists, speech and language therapists, dieticians, restorative dentists and prosthetic specialists.

What are the changes to oral cancer staging in the AJCC/UICC TNM 8th edition (2017)?

For the primary tumour, depth of invasion (DOI) has been recognised as an important prognostic factor with a depth of 5–10 mm upstaging a sub 2 cm primary to T2 and a DOI ≥10 mm automatically making a lesion at least T3. N staging has also been modified with a clinical and pathological staging system, with any extra-nodal extension upstaging the disease. The previous N3 TNM7 category is split into (a) and (b) subcategories depending on the presence of extra-nodal extension.

 Kerawala C, Rocques T, Jeannon J-P et al. Oral Cavity and Lip Cancer: United Kingdom National Multidisciplinary Guidelines; *J Laryngol Otol.* 2016;130(Suppl 2):S83–9.

Oropharyngeal Cancer

LAURA WARNER

Please describe this image

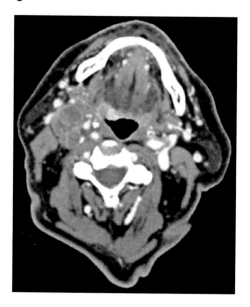

'This is a contrast enhanced axial CT image of the neck, at the level of the oropharynx. The obvious abnormality demonstrated is a cluster of enlarged and necrotic lymph nodes in right level II and there is asymmetry of the tongue base with increased bulk and an area of hyper-enhancement in the right tongue base'.

Important points to cover in the history

- Onset and progression of symptoms: Pain, odynophagia, otalgia
- Onset and progression of neck lump and associated symptoms e.g. pain
- Current nutritional status, weight loss
- Risk factors: Smoking, alcohol intake
- Past medical history, previous head and neck cancer treatment, estimate performance status
- Family/social support

Talk me through your initial management of this patient

After taking a history covering the points previously mentioned you would conduct a full head and neck examination focussing on:

- *Neck nodes*: Are they mobile or do they feel fixed and infiltrative? – this might imply extra nodal extension
- *Assess the oropharynx*: Is there restricted mouth opening which might make intubation difficult or may preclude transoral surgery?
- Assess the location and extent of the primary tumour, assess for involvement of the epiglottis and potential airway compromise.

If you see an obvious tumour it is important to sensitively tell the patient your suspicions so that they understand the need for urgent investigations and they are prepared for the outcome. Ideally involve family members or friends in this part of the consultation.

Next you would arrange for cross-sectional imaging of the head and neck and thorax – either CT or MRI are acceptable for the neck, with a CT of the thorax.

You would also arrange for the patient to have a biopsy (ideally after the scan). For tonsil tumours that are easily accessible transorally this could be done in outpatients, however an EUA is useful if transoral robotic or laser surgery is being considered, so that access and resectability of the tumour can be assessed. If you have seen an obvious primary there is no need for cytology from the neck but if there is any uncertainty about the primary tumour this can be useful.

If the patient has pain it is important to offer him/her appropriate analgesia and if they are struggling to swallow you should arrange for their GP to provide supplements or ask for a head and neck dietician to review them.

Your investigations reveal HPV-related SCC in the right tongue base, staged as T2N2M0. What do you do next?

All new cancer diagnoses are discussed at the head and neck MDT and you should mention this, however the examiners will expect you to be able to discuss treatment options and formulate a plan. It is not acceptable to say that the MDT will decide! Practise a succinct answer to this such as:

'*I would present this case at the head and neck MDT. Treatment options for this patient include transoral surgery (or less likely open surgery – there are some instances in which open surgery is appropriate), neck dissection and adjuvant treatment depending upon the pathology, or primary radiotherapy/chemoradiotherapy. Concurrent chemoradiotherapy would be the most common primary treatment for this disease in the UK. I will involve the patient in the decision-making process and ensure support from all members of the MDT (CNS, SLT, dieticians etc.)*'.

The examiners may ask your preferred treatment option – be prepared to give the reasons for your choice.

What is the significance of the HPV-positive result? How does it change your management?

HPV-related oropharynx SCC has a different tumour biology to non-HPV-related disease and often occurs in younger patients without the traditional risk factors for HNSCC. The survival following treatment is significantly higher for HPV-related tumours. Patients are more likely to present with nodal metastases and asymptomatic primary tumours. Patients require appropriate information on HPV. Currently, the treatment options do not differ between HPV- and non-HPV-related tumours.

 Read this for prognostic information about HPV status – Ang K, Harris J, Wheeler R et al. Human papillomavirus and survival of patients with oropharyngeal cancer; *N Engl J Med.* 2010;363:24–35.

The significance is that prognosis is improved with HPV-related disease (particularly non-smokers), irrespective of the treatment.

There is no current published data from randomised controlled trials to support de-escalation of treatment based on HPV status, however there are studies ongoing.

 Read about the De-ESCALaTE HPV trial and the PATHOS study.

As the majority of HPV-positive patients survive for many years after treatment, the long-term effects of treatment should be considered when deciding upon management and the treatment option with the least long-term morbidity should be offered. Transoral surgery has become increasingly popular over chemoradiotherapy in recent years for this reason, as surgery can reduce the fields and dose of adjuvant radiotherapy and potentially avoid the addition of CT. This reduces the short- and long-term toxicity leading to lower rates of long-term swallowing dysfunction and ORN.

Tell me what you know about the TNM 8 staging?

The UICC TNM staging for oropharyngeal SCC has been updated to account for the improved prognosis of HPV-positive disease. The new staging system was introduced in January 2018 (although is still not widely adopted in the UK). It is based on the results of the ICON-S study.

The important changes are:

- Separate pathological classification of nodal disease in HPV-related disease:
  - *pN1*: 1 to 4 positive lymph nodes
  - *pN2*: 5+ positive lymph nodes
  - These changes downgrade the overall stage of most HPV-positive cancers to reflect the improved survival with HPV-positive disease

- New N3 categories (all HNSCC):
  - *N3a*: Metastasis >6 cm
  - *N3b*: Metastasis with extra-nodal extension (for HPV negative only)
- Changes to the nodal staging for NPC
- Revised definition of T3 thyroid carcinoma

O'Sullivan B, Huang S, Garden A et al. Development and validation of a staging system for HPV-related oropharyngeal cancer by the ICON-S: A multicentre cohort study. *Lancet Oncol.* 2016;17:440–51.

Mehanna H, Beasley M, Evans M et al. Read Oropharyngeal Cancer: United Kingdom National Multidisciplinary Guidelines; *J Laryngol Otol.* 2016;130(Suppl 2):S90–6.

Penetrating Neck Trauma

JASON FLEMING

Are you aware of any methods of classifying neck trauma?

Trauma can be described by the mechanism of injury (low vs. high velocity) or anatomically. The latter involves splitting the anterior neck into three zones: (1) clavicles to cricoid cartilage; (2) cricoid cartilage to angle of mandible; (3) angle of mandible to base of skull.

What are the differences to be aware of between low- and high-velocity injuries?

'*Low velocity injuries are usually the result of stab wounds. The sharp objects inflicting these wounds often have small entry wounds but the underlying soft tissue injury can be significant. In addition, high to low trajectories often put Zone 1 structures more at risk, making haemothorax more likely, as well as brachiocephalic and subclavian vessel injury. In contrast, high velocity injuries are usually due to projectile weapons/gunshot wounds. Whilst handguns can result in small entry and exit wound, as the velocity of the injury increases, there is significantly greater damage to surrounding tissue with a wide field of injury due to shockwave and cavitation effects. Oesophageal, spinal cord and brachial plexus injuries are more common*'.

How do you manage a case of severe neck trauma?

Manage according to ATLS® principles with immediate resuscitation focussed on airway, breathing and circulation. Immediate definite airway intervention in the form of ET intubation or surgical airway may be required in the event of significant airway trauma. Intubation through existing neck wounds has also been described. Rapid identification of life-threatening injuries through primary survey is then performed, looking for definitive indications for imaging and/or immediate surgery. If the patient is stable, secondary survey can then proceed to evaluate severity and extent of additional trauma.

What are the indications for immediate surgical management ('hard signs') in the context of head and neck trauma?

- Pulsatile bleeding
- Airway compromise/stridor
- Expanding haematoma
- Bubbling wound/significant air escape
- Subcutaneous emphysema
- Massive haemorrhage with refractory shock

In patients not requiring immediate surgery, what is your approach to management?

There are inevitably different approaches to managing these patients. However, the traditional approach of exploring all wounds that breached the platysma muscle has now been superseded by the availability and speed of modern imaging protocols. CT angiography has revolutionised trauma management and should now be the mainstay of assessment with the ideal qualities of speed, high resolution and high sensitivity. Subsequent investigations and/or diagnostic procedures can then be tailored to the patient's presentation and suspected injuries e.g. vascular (angiography), laryngo-tracheal (flexible nasendoscopy or bronchoscopy), oesophageal (oesophagoscopy or contrast swallow) or neurological (MRI) injuries.

 A suitable management protocol can be found in Khan AM, Fleming JC, Jeannon JP. Penetrating neck injuries. *Brit J Hosp Med.* 2018;79(2):72–78.

How would you manage a significant vascular injury?

'A trauma patient with significant injury requires the immediate availability of an MDT to optimise their outcome. Ideally these teams would all be available on the patient's arrival, but in some cases injuries only become apparent after the removal of dressings. Haematoma and aneurysm formation may also temporarily cause a cessation in bleeding. The first measure with any active bleeding is direct pressure. Insertion of an 18- or 20- French Foley catheter passed into the wound and inflation for temporary tamponade has also been described. There are topical treatments and newer haemostatic agents that can be applied e.g. tranexamic acid, cellulose polymer agents, haemostatic paste with gelatin and thrombin. However, these are temporising measures before definitive intervention in the event of a significant vessel injury. This may be in the form of surgery, especially for Zone 2 injuries, or angiography and endovascular repair if the patient is stable and the injury is not easily accessible in Zone 1 and 3 injuries'.

What are the most common vessels injured in neck trauma? How would you manage a carotid artery injury?

Re-emphasising ABC management here is not incorrect, although you have likely already used this in a previous answer and a very specific knowledge question has been asked.

The most common significant vessel injury is to the IJV due to its lateral position, large size and thin wall. This can be repaired under direct vision or ligated. Approximately 10% of vascular injuries in penetrating neck trauma will involve a carotid artery. When the patient's long-term neurological status is yet to be determined, every attempt should be made to repair the vessel with early involvement of vascular surgeons. Unilateral carotid sacrifice runs the risk of significant cerebrovascular accident and subsequent functional deficit.

Describe the findings in these images performed on a patient who fell through a glass window:

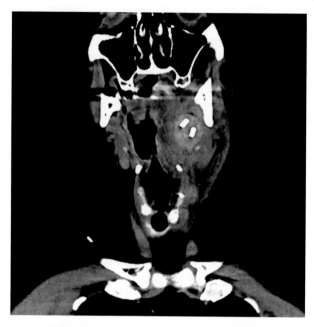

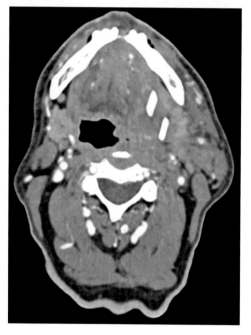

'This is a coronal (left) and axial (right) slice of a contrast CT scan of the neck. There are two visible foreign bodies that have penetrated through the left submandibular space with an associated haematoma but without any obvious active contrast extravasation. The haematoma is resulting in significant mass effect of the supraglottic and pharyngeal airway to the right. In the context of recent trauma, my main concern is to secure a safe airway in the patient so that we can proceed safely to a surgical exploration'.

Pharyngeal Pouch

JAGDEEP VIRK

Please describe this image

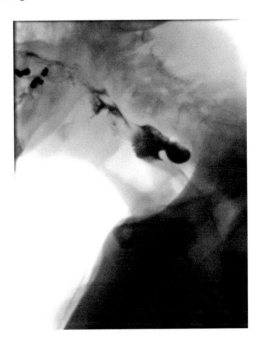

'*This is a contrast swallow demonstrating an outpouching of the pharynx at the level of C4 – 5 consistent with a pharyngeal pouch. It is the length of two vertebral bodies*'.

What is a pharyngeal pouch?

'*A pulsion diverticulum through the pharyngeal mucosa via Killian's dehiscence, a natural weakness between the fibres of cricopharyngeus and thyropharyngeus. The commonest is a posterior diverticulum also called a Zenker's diverticulum*'.

In the vivas, it is important to be ready with succinct definitions. This will allow you to progress to the more challenging or interesting questions. Remember to explain what you (or your centre) would do for this specific patient.

Important elements in the history

 • Patient's age and comorbidities (as these are typically elderly patients, often with potentially difficult endoscopic access)
- Dysphagia
- Loss of weight
- Regurgitation/gurgling
- Halitosis
- Aspiration/pneumonia
- Red flags include dysphonia, neck lump/lymphadenopathy, otalgia

How would you manage this patient?

'*I would take a full history, focussing on the patient's symptomology including weight loss, regurgitation, chest infections, aspiration alongside any red flags and their comorbidities, then go on to examine the patient including flexible nasendoscopy and arrange a contrast swallow*'.

Here it is important to discuss the risks/benefits/alternatives to surgical intervention. This is dependent on the patient's age, wishes, performance status (risk of GA) and symptoms.

What options for intervention are there?

Always remember conservative/non-surgical versus surgical options in answering any question like this.

Conservative for those with few symptoms (e.g. no weight loss or red flags) and/or unfit for GA.

Surgical: Endoscopic or open

 Note: Read NICE guidelines for endoscopic stapling (IPG22).

Endoscopic:

- Stapling

Be able to describe the steps of the procedure including which scopes are used. Remember to inspect the pouch ± biopsy. Consider the patient's teeth – if present, endoscopic stapling can be very challenging.

- CO_2 laser (cricopharyngeal myotomy)
- Diathermy (cricopharyngeal myotomy)
- Botox injection to cricopharyngeus

Open:

- Cricopharyngeal myotomy alone
- Pouch excision and myotomy (diverticulectomy)
- Pouch inversion and myotomy (uncommon)
- Pouch suspension (diverticulopexy) and myotomy
- External pouch stapling

Is the size of the pouch important in deciding your technique? Do you know of any classification system for the pouch size?

Classification systems include Van Overbeek related to vertebral bodies and Morton and Bartley by measurement.

For small pouches, less than 2.5 cm, the endoscopic stapler usually will not fit so other approaches (e.g. CO_2 laser) may be preferable, or an open approach. Similarly, for very large pouches, an open approach may be preferred.

What are the complications of surgery (open and endoscopic)?

- Damage to teeth/gums/lips
- Perforation/mediastinitis
- Revision/failure (10%–20% reported, dependent on approach)
- RLN injury

Post-laryngectomy Care

JASON FLEMING

What do you think are the potential issues for patients recovering from a laryngectomy?

'Recovery and rehabilitation issues can be divided into early and late. Broadly, early factors will be focussed on recovery from the surgery including a period of nil by mouth to allow for anastomosis healing with appropriate alternative enteral or parenteral feeding methods as well as monitoring of the vascularity of any free flap that may have been used for the reconstruction. Once healed, focus will then turn to the recovery of swallowing function and voice restoration, either performed as a primary or secondary procedure. Late factors will focus on follow up for disease recurrence, late onset dysphagia especially in those patients undergoing (chemo)radiotherapy either in the primary or adjuvant setting, as well as ongoing management of the speaking valve in the event of surgical voice reconstruction'.

This is a very broad question. The focus of subsequent questions may depend on how you choose to construct your answer but the examination focus in the post-surgical/rehabilitation scenario is likely to be on speech restoration and dysphagia topics. If there is expectation of more facts, you can go on to mention smoking cessation, nutrition, hypothyroidism management, physiotherapy for any functional deficits after surgery and lymphoedema management.

Describe the speech types available following laryngectomy?

 • Electrolarynx, oesophageal speech, tracheoesophageal speech using voice prosthesis (primary vs. secondary).

What does this photograph show?

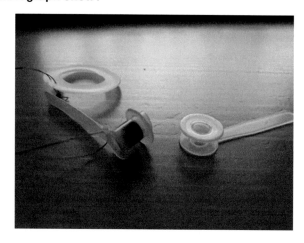

Image credit: Jane Dunton, Acting Clinical Lead Speech and Language Therapist, Head and Neck Oncology, Guy's Hospital, London.

This demonstrates two examples of voice prostheses that are used for surgical voice restoration in laryngectomy patients. Two available brands are shown: Provox (Atos Medical) device on the left with an attached safety medallion and Blom-Singer (InHealth Technologies) on the right. They are produced in a variety of sizes and both clinician-maintained (indwelling) and patient-maintained (ex-dwelling) models are available.

What is primary and secondary voice restoration?

Surgical voice restoration involves creating a puncture site between the posterior tracheal wall close to the laryngectomy stoma and the upper oesophagus. A one-way valve positioned in this tract allows shunting of air into the pharynx when the stoma is occluded. This can be either with a manual or hands-free setup. Key to the quality of this voice is the position and quality of the vibratory segment in the pharyngo-oesophagus in relation to the prosthesis. Primary restoration is performed at the time of the laryngectomy whereas secondary is performed in a delayed fashion following recovery.

> The question of which of these procedures is appropriate for a particular patient is likely above the knowledge required as it depends on a multitude of disease, patient and anatomical factors and is ultimately surgeon specific. A question about this and knowledge that a secondary approach is usually preferable in the post-radiotherapy/salvage setting or if there has been any upper oesophageal resection should ensure a high mark.

What is your approach to valve leakage problems?

The first priority is to ensure prevention of aspiration and you should therefore advise in the event of a significant leak that the patient remains NBM until assessment in conjunction with the speech and language team. Assess whether the leak was through or around the valve.

Central leaks are often secondary to valve failure and therefore cleaning the valve and reassessing, or replacing the valve are both options (in some cases an alternative valve profile type may be required). A swab or direct inspection may confirm Candida colonisation in which case valve replacement and a course of nystatin treatment may be required.

Peripheral leaks may be due to an incorrect length of valve, however if persistent this may indicate a compromised party wall. Fitting progressively larger valve should be undertaken with caution as it may exacerbate the problem. Once recurrent disease has been excluded, measures to encourage stenosis such as down-sizing should be used. Minimal intervention is usually advised but measures such as injection of filler materials around the valve has been described in small case series (*Eur Arch Otorhinolaryngol. 2005 January;262(1):32–4*). Persistent failure usually requires removal of the valve, often with consideration of local reconstruction and augmentation of the party wall. This can be challenging. The removal of the valve may result in spontaneous closure. Simple suturing of the TEP (trachea-oesophageal puncture) often fails due to poor tissue healing. Various options exist to close a problematic TEP including temporalis fascia graft and 3-layer closure, local flaps or free flaps, tracheal resection and re-anastomosis. Manufactured devices do exist to prevent leakage through a widened TEP, and they can be useful in patients in whom surgical intervention fails or who are unable to undergo further intervention.

> Management of problematic TEPs is a common high-level question.

Why do you think head and neck patients are prone to develop dysphagia following treatment?

However you approach this question, make a systematic list to ensure you don't miss the obvious causes. One example would be to list potential treatment complications by region.

- Oral: Trismus, xerostomia, ORN/pain, loss of teeth due to disease/previous extractions, malocclusion following reconstruction.
- Oropharyngeal/hypopharyngeal: Loss of laryngeal framework/epiglottis, stenosis/stricture, inadequate myotomy at the time of surgery, recurrent disease.
- Muscle/soft tissue: Weakness of swallowing musculature from surgical resection, stiffness from scarring/radiotherapy, functional problems following neck dissection, lymphoedema.
- Pre-treatment dysphagia

Tell me about patient-reported outcome measures patient related outcome measures (PROMS) in dysphagia?

'PROMS in dysphagia specifically are tools to measure a patient's own perception of their swallowing function and the impact that any deficit is having on their quality of life. The most commonly used and the one that I am aware of is the MD anderson dysphagia inventory (MDADI) which comprises domains in physical, emotional and functional status'.

Other examples include specific head and neck cancer dysphagia measures e.g. SOAL, and general tools e.g. SSQ and EAT-10. Most institutions use predominantly one measure unless in a research setting so it is acceptable here to mention others to demonstrate your knowledge about alternative tools but it goes without saying, don't say that you have used them if you haven't!

What are the principles of dysphagia management?

The cornerstone of management in these patients is pre-treatment engagement with MDT professionals and an integrated post-treatment rehabilitation programme. As surgeons we need to consider the surgical approach, extent of resection and reconstructive options to minimise dysphagia potential. Early post-treatment swallowing rehabilitation, which can begin even prior to the initiation of oral feeding, are vital to maintain function. A range of other management options exist for more refractory cases including positional manoeuvres, bolus training, biofeedback through specific surgical management for localised pathology e.g. dilatation for stricture. It is important that these complex patients are managed by a specialist MDT.

Post-laryngectomy Complications

ZI-WEI LIU

Questions on post-laryngectomy complications are common in the exam and the practicalities of management are often not covered in standard textbooks.

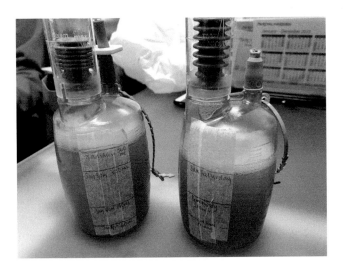

Tell me what you know about chyle leaks after head and neck surgery?

'Iatrogenic chyle leak results from intraoperative injury to the thoracic duct on the left side of the neck as it drains into the postero-lateral aspect of the IJV. However, 10%–25% of chyle leaks may occur on the right due to a high-riding accessory duct'.

What does chyle contain?

Lymphatic fluid and chylomicrons (monoglycerides and fatty acids).

How should chyle leaks be managed?

If a chyle leak is noticed intraoperatively, primary repair should be attempted. Oversewing, application of tissue glue and local muscle flaps have all been described.

Post-operative chyle leaks are divided into low output and high output. Low output chyle leaks drain less than 400 mL/24 hour. These are usually managed conservatively with observation±use of a modified diet. A medium chain triglyceride (MCT) diet is often recommended as this is directly absorbed from the small intestine to the hepatic circulation, bypassing the lymphatic system. Octreotide (somatostatin analogue) has been used as an adjunct.

Intervention is indicated in persistent high output chyle leaks lasting longer than 4–7 days, due to the risk of dehydration, malnutrition or vessel blowout. Re-exploration of the neck is usually the first step, with oversewing, application of tissue glue, mesh or pectoralis major flap. Very rarely intrathoracic ligation of the thoracic duct may be required (thoracic surgery). Transabdominal embolisation has also been described.

What is a pharyngocutaneous fistula?

Pharyngocutaneous fistulas are abnormal connections between the pharyngeal mucosa and the skin surface. Persistent fistula (>4 weeks) increase the risk of vascular erosion.

What risk factors predispose to pharyngocutaneous fistula formation?

Risk factors for pharyngocutaneous fistula formation include previous irradiation, higher tumour stage, extent of surgery (pharyngectomy in addition to laryngectomy), anaemia, hypothyroidism, COPD (chronic obstructive pulmonary disease), and nutritional status. Apart from previous irradiation, other risk factors are not consistently reported across studies. Concurrent chemotherapy and radiotherapy as the primary treatment modality increases the risk of fistula in salvage laryngectomy, compared to radiotherapy alone. Incidence of fistula is reported as between 20% and 60%.

How can pharyngocutaneous fistulas be treated?

Some clinicians advocate free flap or pedicled flap reconstruction of the pharyngeal defect, along with a salivary bypass tubes at the time of surgery for salvage laryngectomy. The addition of unirradiated tissue to augment the pharynx has been shown to reduce fistulae rates.

Pharyngocutaneous fistula can be managed conservatively (NBM, NG/PEG) feeding, use of hyoscine or other saliva suppressants). If conservative measures fail after several weeks or if the fistula leads to severe wound breakdown with risks to the great vessels then surgical intervention can be appropriate. The pec major muscle only flap would be the treatment of choice to cover a fistulae, with free flaps more risky in an inflamed/infected neck. Microvascular anastomoses have a higher failure rate in these settings.

What is the significance of laryngectomy stomal stenosis?

Stomal stenosis post-laryngectomy can impede access to the voice prosthesis. It is rare for stenosis to cause catastrophic airway compromise, but acute presentations can occur.

Early stomal stenosis can be managed by simple dilatation with a laryngectomy tube. A number of techniques have been described for surgical revision, the commonest ones being Z-plasty, V-Y inset±cartilage split. Skin grafts and radial forearm flaps have also been described.

You may be asked to draw one of these flaps so they are worth practising.

V-Y Inset flap

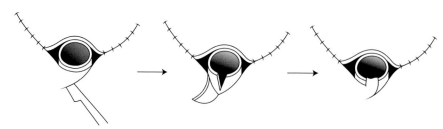

Radiotherapy, Chemotherapy and Osteoradionecrosis

JAGDEEP VIRK

It is important to understand the role of radiotherapy and chemotherapy for head and neck neoplasia, not only for the exam but also in explaining the process/options to patients. It can come up in the viva section and also in the clinical scenarios.

What is radiotherapy and how does it work?

'Radiotherapy is the use of ionising radiation and can be internal (e.g. brachytherapy, radioiodine) or external (e.g. x-ray, gamma ray; particulate – electrons, neutrons, protons). Radiotherapy works by damaging cellular DNA either directly or indirectly (by free radical generation). This ultimately results in cell death'.

In your clinical scenario look closely for scars and post-radiotherapy changes including subtle signs such as telangiectasia. Always check twice in areas where scars heal well (e.g. parotid) and in elderly patients.

Indications for radiotherapy

- Radical radiotherapy: Primary treatment of head and neck malignancies. Rarely benign disease (e.g. carotid body tumour, recurrent pleomorphic adenoma)
- Adjuvant/PORT: Tumour factors and lymph node factors
- High stage primary tumours (T3 and T4)
- Close or involved surgical margins
- Perineural invasion or lymphovascular invasion
- Involved lymph node metastases (single N1 disease can be managed by surgery alone but it would be reasonable to offer adjuvant radiotherapy too – this is debatable and lacking in clear evidence)
- Indications for the addition of chemotherapy in the adjuvant setting are positive margins and ECS

What is the radiotherapy regime in your hospital for T3N0M0 larynx?

60–70 Gy over 30–35 fractions.

Know your local protocols as they differ between centres.

What is a Gray (Gy)?

'The amount of energy in joules absorbed per unit kilogram of matter. 1 Gy =1 J kg⁻¹'.

What are the side effects of radiotherapy?

Consider this question in terms of acute and chronic complications.

Remember the long-term risk of second malignancy (e.g. radiation-induced sarcoma).

Acute: Fatigue, lethargy, mucositis, odynophagia and dysphagia, weight loss, skin damage, aspiration risk.

Chronic: Xerostomia, dysphagia, loss of taste, fibrosis, lymphoedema, dental caries, rarely radiation-induced tumours, carotid artery stenosis and increased risk of stroke, cranial neuropathies.

 Read about fractionation and the benefits of IMRT

What are ORN and pathophysiology?

'An area of non-healing exposed bone for at least three months in a previously irradiated field'.

Pathophysiology includes vascular inflammation and fibrosis secondary to radiotherapy/CRT, leading to tissue hypovascularisation and hypoxic injury, making the area susceptible to necrosis and secondary anaerobic infection.

The mandible is more susceptible in part due to type of bone and also blood supply (particularly the anterior segments). Other risk factors to check in the history are:

- Smoking
- Bisphosphonates
- Local infection/inflammation/dental trauma
- Atherosclerosis
- Diabetes
- Higher dose radiotherapy (possibly less common with IMRT)

How would you manage a patient with mandibular ORN?

Non-surgical versus surgical:

- Non-surgical options include improving nutrition status, smoking cessation, treating infection, controlling risk factors (e.g. diabetes control, stopping bisphosphonates), hyperbaric oxygen (limited evidence), medications (e.g. pentoxyphyline, tocophorol)
- Surgical options exclude recurrence and resect with soft tissue/free flap reconstruction (e.g. fibula)

 Read ENT UK Head & Neck guidelines - Restorative dentistry and oral rehabilitation.

Note the importance of oral/dental review in the peri-treatment phase in preventing oral complications.

When are cells most sensitive to radiotherapy?

Radiotherapy works by damaging DNA of cancer cells. Cancer cells lose cell cycle checkpoint regulation and rely primarily on the G2/M checkpoint having lost G1/S checkpoint control due to the loss of p53. Therefore cancer cells are most sensitive to radiation in G2 and M phase and most resistant in S phase. Molecular targeting of the G2/M checkpoint in conjunction with radiotherapy is being explored as a potential novel therapy.

Please can you describe chemotherapy regimes in head and neck cancer?

Chemotherapy is the systemic therapeutic use of chemical agents to treat disease. It can be classified as induction, concurrent (i.e. chemoradiotherapy) and adjuvant/post-operative (post-operative chemoradiotherapy).

Induction CT: No level 1 evidence for an advantage in using induction regime prior to chemoradiotherapy, but can be considered in primary treatment of NPC and primary treatment of rapidly progressive disease. There may be a role for reducing time to metastatic relapse.

Concurrent chemoradiotherapy (weekly or fortnightly regimes) is the recommended schedule. Here, chemotherapy may have a role in sensitising tumour cells to the effects of radiation. Definite survival advantage. Recent evidence has shown that cetuximab with radiotherapy leads to inferior survival compared to cisplatin and radiotherapy for oropharyngeal cancer (De-ESCALate trial).

Post-operative chemoradiotherapy may be for positive margins and ECS (level 1 evidence), age (or biological age) should be less than 70.

Can you classify the chemotherapeutic agents commonly used in head and neck cancer?

- Platinum-based (commonly cisplatin)
- Pyrimidine analogue antimetabolites (e.g. 5-FU)
- Taxanes (e.g. docetaxel)
- Monoclonal antibodies (this is often used when cisplatin-based CT is contraindicated e.g. renal failure or in platinum refractory disease)

 It is useful to learn mechanism of action and common side effects for Part 1. Chemotherapy agents can be cell cycle-dependent or cell cycle-independent; this helps to plan chemotherapy regimes in terms of timings/doses.

What is the role for planned neck dissection for N2-3 SCC following primary CRT?

 Discuss the PET-NECK study which showed that survival was similar in patients with N2 or N3 head and neck cancer managed by PET-CT surveillance at 12 weeks (with neck dissection if PET-CT showed incomplete or equivocal response) compared to planned neck dissection. In the PET-CT group there were fewer operations and it was more cost effective than planned neck dissection here. Note the paucity of data for N3 subset.

Mehanna H, Wong W-L, McConkey CC et al. PET-CT surveillance versus neck dissection in advanced head and neck cancer. *N Engl J Med*. 2016;374(15):1444–54.

Ranula

CHADWAN AL-YAGHCHI

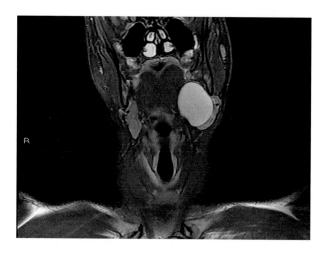

Can you describe the findings in this image?

'This is a T2 weighted MRI in coronal section showing a cystic lesion in the left floor of mouth extending into the left submandibular region displacing the left submandibular gland laterally. This is most in keeping with a plunging ranula'.

Remember, water is bright in T2 images.

What is a ranula?

Ranula is mucus extravasation pseudocyst in the soft tissue of the floor of mouth. This can be caused by obstruction of the sublingual gland duct or trauma, including iatrogenic, to sublingual or submandibular gland or their ducts. Ranulas can herniate through the mylohyoid muscle into the soft tissue of the neck. This is called a plunging ranula and represents around 10% of all ranulas.

Important elements in the history

- Onset, duration, progression
- Salivary gland surgery
- Salivary gland pathology including stones
- Smoking and alcohol history
- Dental history
- Red flag symptoms

What is the differential diagnosis?

 • Lymphangioma (cystic hygroma)
- Haemangioma
- Retention cyst
- Dermoid cyst
- Minor salivary gland tumour

What are the treatment options?

- Aspiration (with or without US guidance) is mainly indicated for symptomatic control of very large ranulas. It carries high risk of re-accumulation.
- Intralesional sclerotherapy under US guidance. Sclerosing agents include OK-432 (Picibanil) which is a lyophilised mixture of a low virulence *Streptococcus pyogenes* incubated with benzylpenicillin.
- Marsupialisation.
- Minimally invasive silk suture technique to obliterate the extravasation site.

 See Professor Mark McGurk's YouTube video of the technique.

- Excision via intraoral, transcervical or combined approach. Excision should include the ipsilateral sublingual gland to reduce the risk of recurrence. Complication includes damage to the lingual nerve and submandibular gland duct.

 Patel MR, Deal AM, Shockley WW. Oral and plunging ranulas: What is the most effective treatment? *Laryngoscope*. 2009;119:1501–9.

Salivary Gland Malignancy

JAGDEEP VIRK

This patient attends your head and neck clinic complaining of a firm lump in her right cheek.

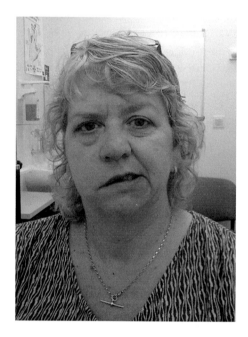

How might this patient present and how would you manage them?

If you are offered an open-ended question, remain systematic and go through relevant aspects of history, examination, investigations (histological/cytological, radiological, bloods, microbiological) and treatment options.

Important elements in the history

 • Onset, duration, progression (rate of change) of lump
  • History of facial weakness or pain
  • Previous surgery (parotid and skin)
  • Other lumps

The patient tells you the mass has grown steadily, they have had neuralgic like right facial pain and now have noticed a facial weakness. How would you proceed?

'In this particular case, there are features in the history suggestive of malignancy. I would explain to the patient that this my concern and proceed to organise cross-sectional imaging. MRI is preferable for delineation of soft tissue structures in the suprahyoid neck and demonstrates the deep lobe (parapharyngeal) component, which would not be apparent on ultrasound. I would request a CT thorax to determine whether there are distant metastasis and an US guided FNA-C or core biopsy for histological diagnosis'.

Please describe this image

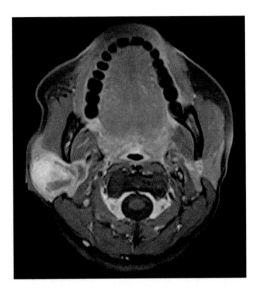

'This is a post-contrast T1 weighted axial MRI through the suprahyoid neck, demonstrating a lobulated right parotid mass extending into the superficial and deep lobes of the gland, with cystic and high signal areas'.

The cytology returns an adenoid cystic carcinoma (ACC). What are the options? What would you recommend?

'This is a malignant epithelial tumour of the parotid gland and this patient should be managed with an MDT approach. There are non-surgical and surgical options. However, I would recommend surgical excision in a patient medically fit enough for a GA. In this case a total parotidectomy is advocated with resection of adjacent structures to ensure an en-bloc resection'.

ACC typically spreads diffusely with frequent perineural spread. Sacrifice of any part of the facial nerve overtly infiltrated with tumour is recommended. A neck dissection should be performed in this case (although some T1N0 ACCs may not require a neck dissection), if there is clinical or radiological evidence of nodal disease. PORT would be indicated for this patient.

What are the complications of surgery?

Bleeding, infection, pain, collection/haematoma, scar, numbness, Frey's syndrome, first bite syndrome, fistula.

Remember to also include facial weakness depending on the patient's pre-operative condition. You may at this point be asked about facial reanimation – intraoperative or delayed. See the Facial Palsy chapter in the otology section.

You should be able to define Frey's syndrome succinctly and provide an explanation for its pathophysiology.

How do you identify the facial nerve?

- Tympanomastoid suture line
- Posterior belly of digastric
- Tragal pointer
- Retrograde dissection (may be useful in this case)

Can you tell me about the common neoplasms of the salivary gland and the rates of malignancy?

- Parotid gland: 80% benign
- SMG: 60% benign
- Minor salivary glands: 50% benign
- Sublingual: 20% benign

Benign lesions are epithelial (pleomorphic adenoma, Warthin's) or non-epithelial (lymphangioma).

Malignant lesions are low (e.g. acinic, low grade mucoepidermoid) or high grade (e.g. adenoid cystic).

For Part 1 in particular, it is worth reading about the basic salivary gland unit, types of cells and related malignancies including TNM stage/differing patterns of spread/basic histology.

Read about management of the facial nerve and the neck/radiotherapy in cases of malignancy. These are areas of debate and may come up in the latter stages of the viva.

Sood S, McGurk M, Vaz F. Read Management of Salivary Gland Tumours: United Kingdom National Multidisciplinary Guidelines. *J Laryngol Otol.* 2016;130 (Suppl. S2):S142–9.

Sialolithiasis

CHADWAN AL-YAGHCHI

A 45-year-old female presented with a 6-month history of recurrent swelling in the right submandibular region.

How would you approach this patient?

Essential elements in history:

- Onset, duration, progression
- Relation to eating
- Infection and antibiotics
- Dental history
- Red flag symptoms
- Smoking and alcohol use
- Systemic diseases (diabetes, HIV and autoimmune conditions)

The patient symptoms started after an acute infection in the area that was treated with antibiotics by her GP. Since then she has suffered recurrent swelling after eating that lasts for few hours.

The most likely cause of the patient symptoms is a submandibular gland stone.

Differential diagnosis:

- Duct strictures
- Mucus plug
- Tumour
- Foreign body

Start with a full ENT examination including digital palpation of the floor of mouth, bimanual palpation of the submandibular gland, full neck examination.

First-line investigation is USS±FNA (fine needle aspiration) biopsy. US may not show the stone but acoustic shadow and duct dilatation can identify the stone location. Similarly, the US may not show a stricture or a mucous plug, however it will help identify (or exclude) any associate pathology such as sialadenitis or tumours.

Be prepared to defend your choice of investigation (US vs. sialoendography). US is readily available, non-invasive with no radiation exposure. While it might miss a stricture or a small stone it will detect parenchymal lesions.

Similarly, if a stone is palpable in the floor of mouth would you arrange an USS or proceed directly to surgical treatment. Stick to what you do in clinic and prepare to be challenged.

Depending on the clinical picture and US findings, the second-line investigation is sialography. This is the gold standard investigation for imaging the submandibular duct and the intraglandular ductal system. It will detect and localise strictures and sialolithiasis. It can be therapeutic as small stones and mucus plugs can be flushed with the contrast. In addition, sialography require dilatation and cannulation of the ductal punctum which can help with the salivary flow. There is a risk of introducing infection with sialography.

Other investigation modalities:

- *MR sialography*: Not widely available
- *Floor of mouth X-ray*: Can miss a radiolucent stone (only 20%–25% are radiopaque)
- *CT scan*: Similarly it can miss a radiolucent stone and cannot localise the stone in relation to the ductal tree
- *MRI scan*: Mainly to further investigate suspected soft tissue pathology

How would you manage an intraductal stone?

Depending on the size and location of the stone (anterior or posterior) and if palpable in the floor of mouth treatment options are:

- *Conservative treatment*: Sialagogues, hydration and manual massage.
- *Medical treatment*: Antibiotics and NSAIDS as indicated.
- *Simple intraoral stone removal*: Can be done under LA in clinic or day surgery. Start by putting a silk suture behind the stone to prevent posterior displacement then make an incision over the stone and extract. Marsupialise the open duct following stone extraction. The risk of recurrent calculi or SMG obstructive symptoms is reasonably high.
- *Sialoendoscopy*: Can be used for small stones up to 4 mm. Larger stones can be broken using pneumatic lithotripsy or can be pulled using a wire basket into the papilla of the duct then proceed as previously detailed. Sialoendoscopy can be used for parotid and submandibular glands and can be done under LA with/without sedation or under GA.
- *Interventional radiology*: The stone is located using contrast then removed with wire basket. Strictures can be balloon dilated.
- Extracorporeal lithotripsy.
- *Salivary gland excision*: Most commonly indicated for recurrent symptomatic submandibular gland calculi. Calculi over 4 mm or calculi situated in the hilum of the gland or within the gland are challenging to manage conservatively. Parotidectomy for recurrent sialolithiasis is complicated by the risk of facial nerve damage within a chronically inflamed gland and post-operative salivary fistulae. It can be indicated following failed conservative management.

Thyroid Pathology

ZI-WEI LIU

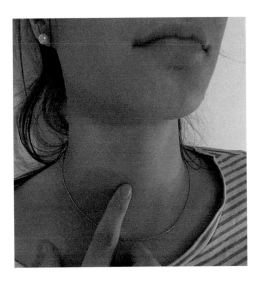

A 36-year-old woman presents with a 6-month history of a right sided thyroid lump. Explain how you would begin assessing this patient.

'I would begin by asking about duration of symptoms/rate of growth/change in voice/difficulty in swallowing/cosmetic issues/airway symptoms. I would also determine whether this patient has any factors for high risk disease: Age (gender, males have a higher risk for poor prognosis in cancer), history of irradiation, family history, autoimmune thyroiditis (predisposes to thyroid lymphoma)'.

What would you look for on examination?

'I would look for previous scars, prominent veins, facial plethora (thoracic inlet obstruction, SVC obstruction). I would listen for hoarse voice and stridor. I would palpate for a central neck mass which moves up and down on swallowing and for lateral cervical lymphadenopathy. If a multinodular goitre is suspected assess for retrosternal extension of the gland by palpating the lower limit. I would perform flexible nasendoscopy to assess for vocal cord movement'.

How would you investigate this patient?

The first-line investigation should be USS neck±FNA as required.

Baseline TFTs and thyroid autoantibodies should be obtained.

Cross-sectional imaging such as CT neck can be indicated for some thyroid malignancies, and for retrosternal goitres to ascertain the lower limit of the goitre.

What is U-grading and Thy-grading?

U-grading is the British Thyroid Association system of grading US nodules which gives an estimate of likelihood of malignancy. Thy-grading refers to the Royal College of Pathologists guidance on the reporting of thyroid cytology specimens.

The nodule is U3 on ultrasound, 2 cm and Thy3f by FNA-c. What would you recommend as next step of management?

This should be discussed at thyroid MDT. A Thy3f nodule carries a 30% risk of malignancy (reported rates of follicular neoplasm vary from 15% to 30%) therefore the MDT would usually recommend diagnostic hemithyroidectomy. Thy3a carries lower risk (10%–15%) of malignancy therefore repeat US surveillance is usually recommended.

The post-operative histology shows a 2 cm follicular carcinoma, completely excised. What would be the next step?

A 2-cm well-differentiated thyroid carcinoma (such as papillary or follicular) can be managed with hemithyroidectomy alone as per British Thyroid Association guidelines.

For tumours between 2 and 4 cm a completion thyroidectomy can be offered but some surgeons will perform hemithyroidectomy alone in young patients. Total thyroidectomy is indicated for cancers over 4 cm.

A completion thyroidectomy is offered to the patient, but you notice on clinical assessment the patient has a vocal cord palsy on the operated side. What would you do?

Delay completion surgery until the vocal cord palsy recovers. If it does not, a pre-operative discussion should be done with the patient with regard to risks of completion thyroidectomy versus US surveillance. A tracheostomy is likely if both recurrent laryngeal nerves are injured.

What is the role of radioactive iodine (RAI) in the management of thyroid cancer?

RAI is offered as adjunct treatment post-surgery for high-risk thyroid cancers on the basis of size of tumour, age of patient, extent of disease (e.g. local or regional metastases). Low-dose RAI is now offered on the basis of the HiLo trial that showed low-dose RAI was as effective as high-dose RAI with fewer side effects. RAI can be given multiple times but there is reduced tumour uptake on repeated exposure. RAI can only be given if a total thyroidectomy has been performed in the cancer setting.

 Further reading:

Mallick U, Harmer C, Hackshaw A. The HiLo trial: A multicentre randomised trial of high- versus low-dose radioiodine, with or without recombinant human thyroid stimulating hormone, for remnant ablation after surgery for differentiated thyroid cancer. *Clin Oncol (R Coll Radiol)*. 2008 Jun;20(5):325–6. doi: 10.1016/j.clon.2008.03.010.

How would you manage a 0.8-cm U5 nodule?

Discuss at the MDT and plan US surveillance for growth. FNA-c is generally not indicated for solitary papillary thyroid carcinoma under 1 cm, and surgery may also not be required. Currently there exists variation in the management of these cases. Multifocal disease would tip the balance towards surgery.

U5 nodules can be medullary carcinoma, which requires surgery regardless of the size of disease, therefore calcitonin is a useful investigation in this setting.

How would you follow up a patient post-treatment for thyroid cancer?

This should be done in the MDT clinic with endocrine and oncology input. Serum thyroglobulin is a sensitive test for patients who have had a total thyroidectomy and RAI ablation and rises with recurrent disease. For patients who have had a hemithyroidectomy US surveillance is preferred.

How would you manage a patient presenting with multinodular goitre?

Multinodular change in the thyroid is extremely common with increasing age and in the majority of cases require no action. Indications for surgical intervention include mass compression of the airway or oesophagus, cosmetic concerns, rapid enlargement (need to check for malignant change, work up as for thyroid nodule).

How would you investigate and treat a multinodular goitre?

If retrosternal extension is suggested on US a CT neck and chest is required. Approximately 5%–10% of retrosternal goitres may need a sternal split undertaken jointly with thoracic surgeons. Factors that increase the likelihood of sternal split include extension of goitre below the aortic arch, narrow thoracic inlet and malignancy.

RAI has very limited indication in multinodular goitre treatment in those who are unfit or unwilling to undergo surgery. It is contraindicated in goitres with airway compression as short-term swelling from RAI may precipitate airway collapse.

 Read the latest British Thyroid Association Guidelines for the Management of Thyroid Cancer. This subject often comes up in Part 1 as well. It is also important to read about dynamic risk stratification of thyroid cancer and its impact on follow up management.

Unknown Primary Cancer in the Head and Neck

LAURA WARNER

Please describe this image

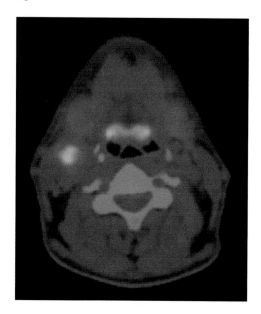

'*This is an axial fused section from a PET-CT scan, at the level of the oropharynx which demonstrates FDG uptake in a right level II lymph node, with symmetrical uptake in the lingual tonsils*'.

What is a PET-CT? How does it work?

A PET-CT scan combines images from PET and CT scans, producing a superimposed functional image. PET scanning is a nuclear medicine imaging modality that uses FDG as a biologically active tracer that is taken up by metabolically active tissues i.e. tumours. The SUV of FDG is calculated and compared to physiological uptake to determine if the area of concern (i.e. a lymph node or lung nodule) are pathological.

How do you think this patient presented? Talk me through your initial management of this patient.

Answer open-ended questions systematically, starting with an overview of what you would do and then give details. The examiners want to see that you have a logical and thorough approach to managing patients presenting with neck lumps.

'*I would expect this patient to have presented with a neck lump. In clinic I would take a history and examine the patient. My history would focus upon... I would conduct a full head and neck examination including fibreoptic nasendoscopy, specifically looking for asymptomatic primary lesions in the nasopharynx, oropharynx or hypopharynx. Next I would arrange investigations...'*

Important points to cover in the history

- Onset and progression of the lump
- Symptoms attributed to the lump i.e. pain, swelling, erythema, discharge, bleeding
- Associated upper aerodigestive tract red flag symptoms: Odynophagia, dysphagia, otalgia, dysphonia
- General symptoms: B symptoms, weight loss, infective symptoms
- Risk factors: Smoking, alcohol intake
- General medical history including any previous head and neck cancer treatment, estimate performance status
- Family/social support

Differential diagnoses for a level II lump:

- Malignant
  - Metastatic SCC: HPV or non-HPV related
  - Lymphoma
  - Salivary malignancy/lymph node metastasis
  - Thyroid metastasis
  - Cutaneous SCC metastasis
  - Lymph node metastasis from non-head and neck primary carcinoma
- Benign
  - Reactive lymphadenopathy
  - Branchial cyst
  - Paraganglioma: Vagal paraganglioma or carotid body tumour
  - Lipoma

Your 45-year-old male patient with a neck lump has no other symptoms or abnormalities on examination. What do you do next?

'I would arrange for the patient to have an USS guided FNA-c or core biopsy and cross-sectional imaging with an MRI of the head and neck and CT thorax. If no primary lesion is seen on imaging and the cytology proves malignancy, then I would request a PET-CT'.

Different institutions use different imaging modalities as standard so tell the examiner what you would do and be prepared to give a reason i.e. I choose MRI over CT for the neck as MRI has better soft tissue definition to detect lesions in the oropharynx. Most units recommend CT or MRI prior to PET-CT as this may detect the primary and are generally cheaper and more accessible.

What are the indications for PET-CT in ENT?

- Unknown primary head and neck SCC
- Staging of lymphoma
- Recurrent head and neck SCC – if considering radical treatment
- T4 hypopharyngeal or nasopharyngeal SCC
- N3 nodal status for any HNSCC

The cytology suggests a benign squamous-lined cyst: What is the most likely diagnosis and what do you do next?

This result suggests a branchial cyst, however in patients over 40 years of age you should still be suspicious that this could represent a metastasis from unknown primary SCC as nodal metastasis from HNSCC are frequently necrotic, particularly HPV-positive disease and this could give similar imaging and cytology findings.

The next step is to ask a head and neck radiologist to repeat the USS, to aspirate the cyst fluid then take a core biopsy from the cyst wall.

If repeat FNA or core biopsy is still negative, cyst excision may be warranted. PET-CT should be considered at this stage as it may detect other findings suggestive of malignancy. The incision should be placed in line with a neck dissection incision so that if revision neck dissection is required the scar could be excised. Consideration should be given to performing a limited level IIa and III neck dissection concurrently if there is a suspicion of malignancy.

Repeat cytology shows p16 positive SCC and the PET-CT shows the level II lymph node but no other areas of abnormal SUV uptake. What is p16?

'P16 is a surrogate marker for high-risk HPV types as HPV-positive cancers overexpress p16 which is a tumour suppressor gene'.

Do you know of any other immunohistochemistry tests that are useful in identifying an occult primary?

Testing for EBV-associated NPC with EBER by in situ hybridisation.

What would you do next?

The next step is to search for the occult primary tumour, which are normally found in oropharyngeal lymphoid tissue.

The patient should undergo panendoscopy including EUA post-nasal space. If there is no visible primary lesion, the tonsils should be removed for histology. In units with transoral robotic or transoral oropharyngeal laser capabilities tongue base mucosectomy may also performed. Alternatively, traditional practice is to take blind biopsies from both sides of the tongue base, although this is much less likely to locate an occult primary.

The results of investigations should be discussed at the head and neck MDT where a treatment plan can be determined. Treatment is likely to entail transoral surgery (if the primary is located) and neck dissection with adjuvant radiotherapy or primary radiotherapy with or without concurrent chemotherapy.

Further reading:

Winter S, Ofo E, Miekle D et al. Trans-oral robotic assisted tongue base mucosectomy for investigation of cancer of unknown primary in the head and neck region. The UK experience; *Clin Otolaryngol.* 2017;42(6):1247–51.

Investigation and management of the unknown primary with metastatic neck disease: United Kingdom National Multidisciplinary Guidelines; *J Laryngol Otol.* 2016;130(S2):S170–5.

Vocal Cord Palsy

CHADWAN AL-YAGHCHI

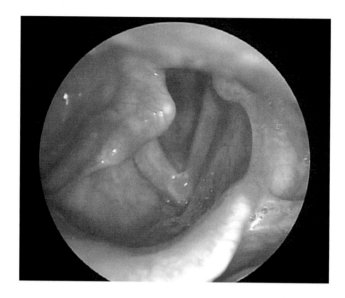

Can you describe the findings in this image? (typically this may be a video in the exam)

'*This is an endoscopic view of the larynx showing unilateral immobile vocal cord on the right. The left cord mobility is normal. There is an anteromedial displacement of the right arytenoid cartilage. The laryngeal mucosa appears healthy with no visible lesions or mucosal changes*'.

Vocal cord immobility is the most accurate term to describe an immobile vocal cord, however you can use the word palsy instead. Avoid using the word paralysis unless a neurological aetiology is confirmed.

Important elements in the history

- Onset, duration, progression of symptoms
- Voice change, aspiration, poor cough, dyspnoea and recurrent chest infection
- Smoking – raises the concern of underlying lung cancer
- Previous surgery (thyroid, cardiac)
- Lung and thyroid tumours
- Intubation history
- Systemic diseases (e.g. RA)

What are the causes of vocal cord immobility?

 Vocal cord palsy:

- Idiopathic
- Post viral infection
- Iatrogenic: Post thyroidectomy or cardiac surgery
- Neoplastic: Lung tumours, thyroid tumours or vagal schwannomas
- Neurological: More likely to be bilateral

Cricoarytenoid joint fixation (rarer):

- Traumatic intubation
- RA
- Posterior glottis scarring

How would you investigate this patient?

- Full examination including neck, thyroid and CNs.
- Videostroboscopy if available.
- CT scan from skull base to diaphragm ('cross-sectional imaging covering the full course of the recurrent laryngeal nerve').

CXR is also an option as it can be done immediately, however it will miss neck lesions and small lung and mediastinal tumours.

Other investigations to consider, following a normal CT scan, are as follows:

- Video fluoroscopy to assess swallowing and aspiration risk especially in vagal nerve injury rather than recurrent laryngeal nerve.
- EMG can distinguish between paralysis and vocal cord fixation. It can give further information on spontaneous recovery and synkinesis. However, it rarely changes management decision, so it is not widely used.

How would you manage this patient?

Management approach depends on the patient symptoms, onset and aetiology. For example, a patient with a sacrificed recurrent laryngeal nerve during thyroid surgery would benefit from early vocal cord injection medialisation.

There is good evidence to support early injection regardless of aetiology. It is associated with better long-term voice outcomes and patients are less likely to require open medialisation.

Wait and see in an asymptomatic patient especially if likely to recover i.e. an intact stimulating nerve at the end of thyroid surgery.

Speech and language therapy referral for voice and swallowing therapy: Various techniques can be used to reduce the risk of aspiration such as chin tuck, head turn and diet modification.

If patient is still symptomatic and no recovery of function, then vocal cord medialisation either injection or open is performed.

What are the surgical options?

Injection medialisation either as an outpatient procedure under LA or under GA. Injection under LA can be trans-cricothyroid, trans-thyrohyoid or per oral.

Open medialisation (type 1 Isshiki thyroplasty). This should be ideally done under LA with or without sedation. This will allow intraoperative voice feedback. Implant position can be confirmed with flexible nasendoscopy. Implant options are silastic block carved to measure, prefabricated Montgomery implants, titanium plate and Gore-Tex®.

Other surgical options:

- Arytenoid adduction: Technically challenging
- Non-selective laryngeal reinnervation: Ansa cervicalis to recurrent laryngeal nerve

 Heathcote K, Ismail-Koch H, Marie J.-P, Bon Mardion N. An update on laryngeal reinnervation. *ENT Audiology News* 2018;27(2).

What injection materials do you know?

Temporary materials:

- Hyaluronic acid: Can last up to 3 months
- Calcium hydroxyapatite: Lasts around 12 months

Permanent materials:

- Bioplastique: Poor voice outcomes but still in use.
- Fat injection: Less predictable as prone to resorption so you need to over inject but it can be permanent. Coleman technique can improve predictability.

How would you approach differ if the patient had bilateral palsy?

In bilateral vocal cord palsy the main concern is the airway. Depending on the onset and severity of symptoms the patient may require a definitive airway via a tracheostomy under LA or GA. Voice and swallowing are less likely to be affected.

Once the airway is secured and investigations are completed as appropriate the patient can be offered surgical treatment to allow decannulation. Options are:

- Laser arytenoidectomy: Posterior cordotomy is an alternative option, however it is associated with worse voice outcomes.

- Arytenoid suture lateralisation.
- Bilateral selective reinnervation: Only practised in one centre in the UK and only a handful worldwide.
- Laryngeal pacing: Currently only in clinical trials.

Primary laser arytenoidectomy or laser cordotomy instead of tracheostomy is an option. However, you need to demonstrate safety for the exam. If you decide to include this as a treatment option, you need to explain that you considered tracheostomy and that you have experience with the procedure and can perform it safely. Transoral techniques for bilateral vocal palsy may be an option for patients with insidious onset of symptoms e.g. neurological causes.

COMMON OTOLOGY VIVA TOPICS

EDITED BY JAMES R TYSOME AND NEIL DONNELLY

6

- Air conduction hearing devices
- Benign paroxysmal positional vertigo
- Bone conduction hearing implants and middle ear implants
- Cerebellopontine angle tumours
- Cholesteatoma
- Chronic otitis media
- Cochlear implantation
- Ear drops and anaesthetics
- Facial palsy
- Ménière's disease
- Necrotising otitis externa
- Noise-induced hearing loss
- Non-organic hearing loss
- Ossiculoplasty
- Otosclerosis
- Paraganglioma
- Pre-auricular sinus
- Sensorineural hearing loss, presbyacusis, autoimmune hearing loss
- Sudden sensorineural hearing loss
- Temporal bone fracture
- Tinnitus
- Vertigo

Air Conduction Hearing Devices

JAMEEL MUZAFFAR AND SUSAN EITUTIS

Hearing rehabilitation could come into discussion in almost all otology vivas so it is worth having a good grasp of the options. A good working knowledge of air conduction aid options is easy to overlook.

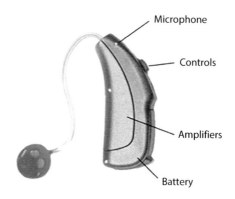

Image credit: John Wills

'*This is a clinical image of a conventional BTE air conduction hearing aid. This is a modern digital aid; though older analogue devices are still in use. The main components are the microphone, amplifier, receiver, manual controls, such as on/off and volume and battery. Sound is detected by a microphone where acoustic energy is converted into electrical energy. This is then processed and amplified before the receiver transforms the amplified electrical signal back into an acoustic signal which is reproduced by the speaker in the patient's ear canal*'.

What types of air conduction hearing aids do you know?

Air conduction aids can be classified into a number of ways. These include analogue or digital, or the style of the device. BTE hearing aids are the most commonly used type with custom aids like ITE, ITC and CIC aids providing arguably improved cosmetic appearance, though sometimes at the cost of more restricted performance options. Custom aids (which are typically not provided in the NHS) can provide very good performance but are limited by the size of the patient's ear canal and are suitable only for patients with a mild to moderate loss. Body worn aids are rarely used now but they allow high levels of amplification and can be suitable for older patients or those with reduced dexterity. CROS aids use a microphone in the worse hearing ear to detect sound which is transmitted wirelessly to the other aid and played into the better hearing ear by air conduction. BiCROS aids function in a way similar to a CROS aid but the better hearing ear is also aided by a microphone on the ipsilateral side.

What is an extended wear hearing aid?

'*An extended wear hearing aid is a type of air conduction aid that is placed deep in the ear canal and can be left in place for up to four months. They are potentially suited to patients with mild to moderate hearing loss and must be placed by an appropriately trained ENT surgeon or audiologist. The main benefit is that the devices cannot be seen without detailed examination of the ear canal, providing excellent cosmesis. Their position is claimed to provide an overall increase in gain and output as well as reduced occlusion effect, reduced feedback and improved directionality*'.

Air conduction aids are commonly used in adults and children to treat sensorineural, mixed or conductive losses as well as tinnitus. These have the advantage that that they are readily available, inexpensive and easy to repair and replace. Contraindications include absent pinna or canal, recurrent infections when wearing aids or thresholds too poor to aid.

As a rule of thumb thresholds worse than 30 dB will benefit from aiding.

BTE hearing aids are the most common hearing aids provided through the NHS and can be used to fit a wide range of hearing losses. BTE aids come in a variety of different receiver strengths with different types of coupling (ear mould/dome) that can be modified based on a patient's individual need. Between 30 and 50 dB open fit varieties are usually employed. These have a small flexible dome that is placed in the canal making them comfortable and quick to fit as they do not require a custom mould of the canal. As hearing losses become more severe, more occluding domes are available to limit the amount of feedback and reduce the amplified sound lost through vents. Thresholds worse than 50 dB usually require an occlusive mould. These improve amplification but reduce ventilation of the ear canal resulting in an increased risk of wax impaction and otitis externa. Aids should be left out if the ear is infected. For patients who do experience recurrent infections/pain from ear moulds, modifications to materials (e.g. soft vs. hard, hypo-allergenic) or widening of vents along with proper cleaning and maintenance may help to reduce these symptoms.

What accessories are available to improve benefits of air conduction digital hearing aids?

Streaming accessories which connect to Bluetooth devices, such as mobile phones, allow a listener to send the audio signals to their hearing aids. This effectively creates a hands-free headset for phone calls and eliminates the need for headphones when listening to music/videos. Remote microphones are also available and enable a listener to better hear someone who is at a distance or in poor listening environments. Remote microphones work by placing a microphone on the speaker's collar; their voice is picked up by the microphone and sent to the hearing aid either directly or via the streamer.

Terms you may be asked to define:

- *Acoustic gain*: The difference in output from the aid compared with input. For example, a tone presented at 50 dB and output at 80 dB would have an acoustic gain of 30 dB.
- *Distortion*: The altered reproduction of sound by a hearing aid.
- *Occlusion effect*: Occurs when an object fills the outer portion of the EAC. This causes the subject to perceive the sound of their own voice as 'hollow' or 'booming'. It is thought to be caused by bone conduction as sounds vibrate back towards the TM from the medial portion of the occlusive object. The effect can increase the sound pressure of low-pressure sounds (typically below 500 Hz) by up to 20 dB. The effect can be reduced by increasing the size of vents and/or the use of hollow tips/domes.
- *Saturation sound pressure level*: The maximum amount of sound pressure (power) that the aid can produce.

Benign Paroxysmal Positional Vertigo

NICHOLAS DAWE

BPPV has a very characteristic presentation with a specific and effective treatment. It is the most common cause of vertigo, with the history central to guiding both the approach to examination, and the decision as to whether further tests might be indicated. Emphasise that you would review the history, if not already provided, and impact of the symptoms on the individual.

Any variation to the characteristic BPPV presentation must be acknowledged. The neurotological exam would be expected to be normal, and imaging is not indicated unless the presentation is unusual. However, BPPV may also coexist with other disease processes such as Ménière's disease and vestibular schwannoma. Patient concerns should be elicited to explore any patient expectations; this might include patient expectations of brain imaging.

What are the theories behind BPPV?

Canalithiasis: 'Otoconia remain loose within the endolymph; this supports both the latency of onset and short duration of symptoms'.

Cupulolithiasis: 'Otoconia attach themselves to the cupula; this links to the symptoms of prolonged vertigo and generalised disequilibrium'.

What forms of BPPV are you aware of?

- Posterior canal canalithiasis >> Posterior canal cupulolithiasis > Lateral canal canalithiasis > Lateral canal cupulolithiasis > Superior canal canalithaisis
- Multicanal BPPV
- Bilateral BPPV

Posterior canal BPPV, followed by lateral canal BPPV, account for the vast majority of cases. Having a robust approach to the assessment, expected findings on positioning tests and options for management would give increased confidence when approaching a viva.

Important elements in the history

- Vertigo: Get the patient to describe the character, onset, precipitating factors
- Ask for any otological history (associated hearing loss, tinnitus, otalgia, discharge, autophony), previous ear surgery, infections, family history
- Impact on life and work (always establish occupation), concerns and expectations of the patient
- Falls in elderly patients/symptoms if sedentary

What are the causes of/risk factors for BPPV?

- Idiopathic (approximately 1/3)
- Previous canal repositioning manoeuvres (a lateral canal BPPV resulting from the treatment of posterior canal BPPV)
- Head trauma
- Whiplash injuries
- BPPV is linked to several inner ear pathologies (Ménière syndrome, vestibular neuritis, SSNHL, otosclerosis and post-stapes surgery)
- Vitamin D deficiency (recurrent BPPV), hypocalcaemia, osteoporosis

Idiopathic BPPV is more common, with a lifetime prevalence of 2.4%. An advancing age brings degeneration of otoconia within the vestibule. It is worthwhile to consider risk factors and associated conditions, particularly for the recurrent and persistent cases.

What is the relevance of the examination to a diagnosis of BPPV?

A diagnosis of isolated BPPV requires that the remaining neurotological exam is normal, and pure tone audiometry should show symmetrical bone conduction thresholds. This serves to exclude a central cause (demyelinating and CNS pathology).

The differential diagnosis of a positional vertigo can be considered according to a central or peripheral origin.

- *Peripheral*: Postural hypotension, vestibular hypofunction, superior canal dehiscence syndrome
- *Central*: Vestibular migraine, central cerebellar vertigo

What are Frenzel glasses?

'*These are goggles with a combination of multiple lenses and a light for viewing the eyes. They allow nystagmus to be easily observed and magnified, whilst at the same time, removing the patient's ability to fixate*'.

How would you assess for posterior canal BPPV?

'*I would perform a Dix–Hallpike examination in any patient presenting with positional symptoms of vertigo. If this was positive – an up-beating nystagmus with a torsional geotropic element (superior pole of the eye towards the affected ear), I would proceed to an Epley manoeuvre, having first counselled the patient and excluded any cervical spine problems*'.

Posterior canal BPPV and the Dix–Hallpike/Epley

Posterior canal BPPV is the most common form of BPPV. The Dix–Hallpike is considered a helpful, though not a highly sensitive test, and a negative test does not rule out BPPV.

If the Dix–Hallpike is negative but subjective symptoms are reported, it is helpful to consider if you should offer Brandt-Daroff exercises, other self-delivered habituation exercises, and/or a formal vestibular assessment that includes VNG. Brandt-Daroff exercises were developed for cupulolithiasis theory of posterior canal BPPV.

The Epley manoeuvre is a highly effective treatment for posterior canal BPPV, however, it can precipitate a lateral canal BPPV in 6%. This means an awareness of features of both posterior- and lateral-canal BPPV are essential.

What tests are you aware of that can confirm other variants of BPPV?

The approach to assessing BPPV relies on positioning tests that are based on Ewald's law (this is simply that the nystagmus should occur in the orientation of the canal being stimulated). Be prepared to deliver a clear statement on how to perform the more common and recognised manoeuvres (Dix–Hallpike or Supine Roll Test).

- *Posterior canal*: Dix–Hallpike. Torsional in the vertical plane upward, torsional, geotropic (towards the affected downmost ear).
- *Lateral canal*: Dix–Hallpike can be used, but ideally the Supine Roll Test (also referred to as the Pagnini-McClure manoeuvre), or the bow and lean test.

Nystagmus is horizontal, and either geotropic (towards the ground) or apogeotropic (away from the ground), depending on whether the debris is within the long arm or short arm of the canal, respectively, as well as, which ear is downmost and therefore being stimulated.

Always observe the eyes on repositioning the head, as the nystagmus reverses and is less intense.

Anterior/superior canal: Dix–Hallpike. It is best to acknowledge that it is extremely uncommon and can be difficult to diagnose. You would expect to see a down-beating nystagmus with more discrete torsional component, occurring with relatively less intensity than occurs in posterior canal BPPV. Such is its rarity, any down-beating nystagmus warrants imaging to exclude a central cause.

What recommendations can you give on the natural history?

BPPV typically has a natural history of resolution, may self-resolve, but recurs in up to 25%.

Canalith repositioning manoeuvres (CRMs) are effective, though cupulolithiasis may be more resistant. BPPV following head injury can also be more resistant to treatment.

What CRM would you perform?

Repositioning manoeuvres reposition the canaliths to the utricle where they are thought to be absorbed. Cupulolithiasis is considered a more resistant form to treatment, and specific CRMs have been designed to target this form of BPPV, such as the Semont manoeuvre. As there are no standardised CRM, however, highlighting the range of those offered and having an answer for most commonly used options is recommended.

- Posterior canal:
  - Epley
  - Semont (liberatory manoeuvre), considered less effective in the longer term, but tends to be used after a failed Epley as may better tackle cupulolithiasis
- Lateral canal:
  - BBQ roll/360° yaw rotation
  - Gufoni manoeuvre

Is there any role for post-manoeuvre recommendations?

There is limited evidence that post-CRM positioning recommendations influence outcome, and no evidence of value of vibratory devices during manoeuvres. When discussing how to perform the positional tests and positioning manoeuvres, emphasise any limitations due to patient factors. Brandt-Daroff exercises alone are effective in only 24% at 3 months when compared to CRMs. There is no evidence to support advising patients to sleep upright for 48 hours. Consider checking Vitamin D levels in recurrent BPPV.

When should a patient with suspected BPPV have an MRI?

- Atypical nystagmus not fulfilling Ewald's law
- Central signs
- Persistent vertigo despite treatment

If an MRI is normal, consider migraine or drugs as a cause.

What is the role of surgery?

The role of surgery is supported by low level evidence in published studies, but it is known to be effective for a minority of persistent (10%) or recurrent (12.5%) cases. It would be best to emphasise that any surgery would be considered after an extensive workup undertaken in a specialist centre, due to risks involved. Surgery consists of posterior semicircular canal occlusion – risks include transient unsteadiness/persisting imbalance, persisting symptoms/late failure, hearing loss (may be anything from a transient mixed loss up to a mild/severe loss in <10%), tinnitus, and facial nerve injury. Both singular neurectomy and vestibular neurectomy are more historical approaches for BPPV.

In recurrent symptoms, performing the appropriate CRM can be effective in up to 98% of cases.

Bone Conduction Hearing Implants and Middle Ear Implants

JAMEEL MUZAFFAR AND JOSEPH MANJALY

What type of device is illustrated in this photograph?

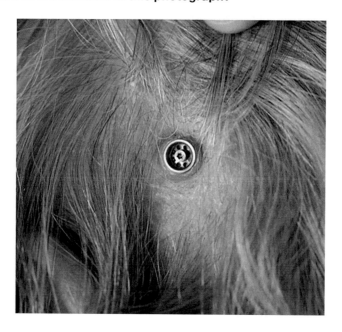

'*This is a photograph of an abutment for use with a bone anchored hearing aid. A titanium fixture is placed into bone and the abutment shown screws into this. A sound processor clips on to that abutment*'.

What types of bone conduction hearing devices are there and how do they work?

The most commonly used systems are percutaneous devices like the system in the picture. These involve the surgical placement of a titanium fixture into bone. Due to osseointegration, vibration from the attached sound processor is transmitted into the skull and through bone conduction to the cochlea. The main drawback of this type of device is skin problems around the titanium abutment. Transcutaneous devices have been designed primarily to reduce skin issues. These systems typically use a permanently implanted component underneath the skin and an external component that is attached by magnetic force. An induction loop is used to transmit the signal to the implant. Other systems include bone conductors worn on a headband or attached by sticky plasters.

With percutaneous devices, the transmission across the skin is 'passive' as the external hearing aid is the only active component. Transcutaneous devices can pass sound passively through the skin or be 'active' with an internal vibrating actuator.

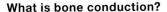

What is bone conduction?

'*Bone conduction is the process through which vibrations are transmitted through the bones of the skull to stimulate the cochlea. It forms a normal part of hearing and can be used to bypass the normally preferential route of air conduction transmission via the EAC, TM and ossicles*'.

What is osseointegration?

'*Osseointegration is a functional ankylosis where new bone is laid down directly onto the implant surface integrating it into the bone resulting in mechanical stability. It is a dynamic process where the characteristics of the implant lead to fusing with surrounding bone through direct contact. The most commonly used material is titanium due to its high tensile strength, corrosion resistance and biocompatibility. It is widely used in dental and orthopaedic surgery as well as in ENT for most bone conducting hearing systems and attachment of prosthetic ears*'.

Terminology around bone conducting hearing devices can be complex. Whilst they are often called BAHA (short for bone anchored hearing aid) this term is a trademark of Cochlear, one manufacturer of such devices. Other manufacturers often term their products bone anchored hearing implant/instrument (BAHI) or bone anchored hearing system (BAHS). Generically, they can be termed 'bone conduction hearing implants (BCHIs)'.

What are the indications for a bone conduction hearing device?

- Conductive or mixed hearing loss. In patients with a large air-bone gap, a BCHI may provide a better result than an air conduction aid.
- Single-sided deafness (consider CROS or BiCROS as an alternative)

Any indication that would be suitable for a conventional air conduction aid but in which the patient is unable to wear one. There are some caveats to this, the main one being that the fitting range is limited to mild-moderate losses. Beyond this range devices typically do not provide enough power. This would include absence or malformation of the pinna or canal, recurrent infections or patients who have had surgery for chronic ear disease with anatomy that makes it difficult to fit a conventional aid. It should also be noted that with transcutaneous devices, skin creates 10–15 dB attenuation as compared to percutaneous devices. Evidence suggests active transcutaneous BCHIs perform better at medium and high frequencies compared to passive devices.

They are particularly useful for conductive hearing losses (CHLs), especially if bone conduction thresholds are significantly better than air conduction and patients are gaining insufficient benefit from an air conduction device.

What are the complications of bone anchored hearing implant surgery?

'*The most common complication is skin irritation, poor wound healing and/or infection, though this is greatly reduced with modern techniques that involve small linear incisions or punches for access and avoid the need to thin soft tissue and apply skin grafts. Other complications include early or late fixture loss as well as bleeding, haematoma and persistent pain*'.

 Read about Holgers scoring system for bone anchored hearing aid skin reactions.

At what age would you consider a bone anchored hearing device in children and why?

'Children can wear a bone conducting device on a soft or hard headband from any age. Surgical fixture placement is usually delayed until the age of four or five years to allow the bone of the skull to thicken to approximately 4 mm. This reduces the risk of failure of osseointegration and subsequent fixture loss. All children considered for fixture implantation should have a trial of a device on a headband first. In adults, it is common to complete the procedure as a single stage operation, often under LA. Children may have surgery as a one or two stage procedure depending on age and thickness of the skull'.

Are there any special concerns when siting osseointegrated fixtures in children with microtia?

'Children will often be considered for a percutaneous hearing solution at the age of around five, much younger than the typical age for autologous ear reconstruction which is often offered at around age ten. Reconstruction usually involves skin flaps from the post-auricular area and discussion within a multidisciplinary setting (ENT, plastic, maxillofacial surgeons and prosthesist) is recommended to avoid siting the fixture in a position where it will limit potential future reconstructive options'.

Questions on bone conducting hearing systems are very common in the FRCS(ORL-HNS), particularly in the clinical stations. Patients are readily available, generally well and have obvious clinical signs to discuss. With this in mind, make sure you are comfortable with the range of auditory implants (BAHI/ bone anchored hearing system (BAHS), middle ear implants (MEIs), cochlear implants [CI] and auditory brainstem implants [ABI]). This is a constantly changing field, with new devices being developed year by year and indications and criteria also rapidly evolving. Therefore, be sure to review recent literature reviews and manufacturer's websites during your exam year.

At the time of publication, these are the most commonly used bone conduction implants in the UK:

- Percutaneous: Cochlear BAHA Connect and Oticon Ponto
- Transcutaneous passive: Cochlear BAHA Attract and Medtronic Sophono (powered component outside skin)
- Transcutaneous active: Med-el Bonebridge (powered component under skin)

Bone conduction devices are able to stimulate both inner ears simultaneously utilising the low attenuation of bone conduction, making them useful in cases of single-sided deafness to overcome the head shadow effect. Note the distinction between these devices and active MEIs, such as the Med-el Vibrant Soundbridge and Cochlear Carina, which *unilaterally* augment middle ear function by directly vibrating the ossicles (or round window).

What is the role of Middle ear implant in the treatment of hearing loss?

MEI are currently a niche area of otology and it is therefore unlikely you will be given a whole viva on the subject. However, the field is rapidly evolving and it is envisaged that expanded capabilities will mean a wider adoption of the technology. An understanding of the current devices and their application is therefore important in any hearing loss viva.

MEIs provide mechanical stimulation via a transducer to the ossicular chain or less commonly, directly to the inner ear fluid. These devices are suitable for patients with mild to severe sensorineural hearing loss as well as conductive hearing loss and mixed hearing loss. The purely unilateral stimulation of MEIs brings subsequent benefits of improved sound localisation and cortical stimulation in addition to improved speech perception in background noise.

One should first consider whether hearing can be improved sufficiently with canalplasty/ tympanoplasty/ossiculoplasty/stapes surgery or an air conduction hearing aid. Consider MEI in cases where this is not possible and hearing is stable and not poor enough to warrant cochlear implantation. Common examples include external and middle ear atresia, external ear canal fibrosis, chronic otitis externa and previously failed middle ear reconstruction surgery.

A minimum threshold of inner ear hearing is required to be able to benefit from the amplification provided by MEIs. Hearing should be stable rather than progressive. The middle ear should be free of disease.

 Review the manufacturer's websites for latest guidelines on audiometric criteria for currently available devices.

At the time of writing, current devices used in the NHS are the Med-el Vibrant Soundbridge and the Cochlear Carina. The Vibrant Soundbridge is able to couple to the ossicular chain via the incus short process but can also couple to the incus long process, the stapes head or directly to the round window depending on the accessibility and availability of middle ear structures (guided pre-operatively by a CT scan). This makes it suitable for hearing amplification in both sensorineural hearing loss and conductive/mixed hearing loss (there are different audiometric criteria for each category). It has an external processor which links via magnet.

The Carina is a fully implanted device that connects to the ossicular chain via an actuator which provides mechanical vibrations. The Carina's internal microphone and processor are implanted under the skin and the external processor is optional depending on the degree of hearing loss. This solution is suitable for patients unable to wear conventional hearing aids or who want a totally implantable solution with no external processor. Battery life and the efficacy of the implanted microphone are the key factors for this class of device in the future.

Cerebellopontine Angle Tumours

NISHCHAY MEHTA

Please describe this image

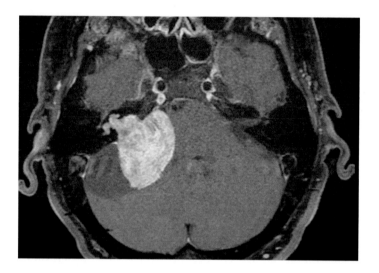

'This is an axial T1 MRI scan with contrast at the level of the temporal bones. There is a large mass arising from the right internal auditory meatus into the CPA. The IAM has been expanded by the mass and there is contrast enhancement within the cochlea and vestibule. The extrameatal component of the tumour is compressing the cerebellum, middle cerebellar peduncle and brainstem with distortion of the fourth ventricle: It is possible that this might have resulted in raised ICP. There looks to be a cyst at the posterior aspect of the mass indicating a cystic component or retained CSF, this would be better evaluated with a T2 scan'.

It is important to be able to evaluate and describe axial MRIs of the internal acoustic meatus. The weighting of the scan can be defined by the colour of the orbit, which if bright, suggests T2 weighted image. Radiolucent orbits with bright blood vessels (either carotid centrally or sigmoid sinus laterally) suggests T1 weighting with contrast. The vestibulocochlear nerves should be traced from brainstem to cochlea.

What do you think is the diagnosis?

'The most common CPA tumour is a vestibular schwanomma accounting for more than 80% of cases. Differentials include meningioma, epidermoid cyst and metastatic lesions'.

Imaging can help differentiate the diagnosis. Vestibular schwanommas are centred on the IAC and are hypointense on T1 and T2 but bright on T1 with contrast. Meningiomas have similar enhancement characteristics but have broad-based tails and are eccentrically positioned on the IAC. An epidermoid cyst is bright on T2 and does not enhance with contrast.

What are vestibular schwanommas and how do they present?

'A vestibular schwanomma is a benign tumour of the Schwann cells and occurs most commonly at the junction of centrally myelinating cells (oligodendrocytes) and peripherally myelinating cells (Schwann cells) at the medial end of the IAC. More than 95% are sporadic whilst 5% are due to autosomal dominant neurofibromatosis type 2'.

The most common presenting symptom is asymmetrical sensorineural hearing loss, tinnitus, and vertigo. Clinical findings are variable and depend on the size of the tumour and may include hearing loss, nystagmus, a peripheral vestibulopathy and CN abnormalities such as reduced facial sensation and rarely, lower CN deficits and signs of raised ICP. Reduced sensation can be noted on the posterior ear canal wall (Hitselberger's sign): This is a common exam question but of relatively little clinical value!

What are the principals of management?

Management should be through a multidisciplinary skull base team, taking into account patient choice. Treatment options include:

- Conservative management with serial scanning: 'Watch, wait, rescan'
- Single fraction (gamma knife) or fractionated (Linac) radiotherapy
- Surgical (mid-cranial fossa, retrosigmoid and translabyrinthine approaches with excision or debulking)

The majority of vestibular schwanommas will never lead to debilitating or life-threatening consequences: At presentation there is a 60% chance that the tumour will not demonstrate any further growth. Surveillance scanning allows the team to differentiate those that will need intervention from those that can be safely monitored without treatment.

Stereotactic radiosurgery is generally considered for non-cystic, growing tumours in patients with tumours less than 2.5 cm maximal intracranial diameter, or without significant brainstem compression. Where there is more brainstem compression, fractionated radiotherapy can be used. Abnormal growth is generally considered as >2 mm per year. The long-term outcomes are still relatively unknown and the risk of radiation-related secondary tumours is a possibility (1% per decade of developing a benign or malignant tumour as a result of having had radiotherapy), as such, there is careful MDT consideration regarding the use of radiotherapy in the young.

Surgery can be considered for larger tumours (>2.5 cm) when they are growing or causing compressive symptoms. For tumours over 2.5 cm, the access would be via a translabyrinthine or retrosigmoid approach depending on individual Skull Base Unit preference. Smaller tumours may be operated on at patient's request or for consideration of hearing preservation where there is good hearing and speech audiometry and where there is CSF (cerebrospinal fluid) lateral to the tumour. Hearing preservation approaches are retrosigmoid or middle cranial fossa.

Vestibular schwannoma in a patient under 30 years old should make the clinician think about neurofibromatosis type 2. This condition features bilateral vestibular schwannomas as well as posterior subcapsular cataracts, spinal tumours and skin lesions. Inheritance is autosomal dominant via a variant in the *NF2* gene on chromosome 22 that encodes the protein Merlin. New mutations can occur, and an estimated 50% patients have no family history. Genetic testing and annual surveillance MRI scanning from childhood are important for anyone with a family history. Specialist MDT management is undertaken in quaternary centres in the UK and ABI is considered in appropriate patients.

 Read about the use of Avastin in NF2 patients.

Cholesteatoma

NICHOLAS DAWE

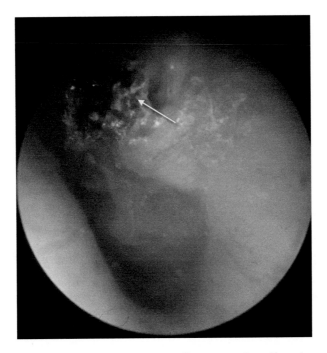

Image credit: Welleschik • CC BY 2.5. https://commons.wikimedia.org/

'*This is an endoscopic photograph of a left ear demonstrating a left attic cholesteatoma*'.

In addition to examining your elective management of cholesteatoma, a case may be presented as chronic otitis media with an acute intracranial complication, whereupon the management of the acute problem is first addressed and thereafter, the principles of cholesteatoma management may be discussed in the remaining part of the viva.

Define a cholesteatoma

'*Cholesteatoma is a mass of keratinising squamous epithelium in the tympanic cavity and/or mastoid with accumulation of keratin debris that can be associated with surrounding inflammation. This is typically explained to the patient as "skin in the wrong place"*'.

Congenital (primary) cholesteatoma is present from birth (persistence of the foetal epidermoid formation in the middle ear), all other cholesteatomas are acquired (secondary). A congenital cholesteatoma is based on the appearance of a white mass in the middle ear, an intact TM and no prior surgery or aural discharge.

There are a number of theories relating to the development of acquired cholesteatoma including:

- Retraction pocket theory (most accepted)
- Basal cell hyperplasia
- Immigration of squamous epithelium through a perforation
- Squamous metaplasia

Be able to offer a classification system for retraction pockets e.g. Tos (pars flaccida) and Sadé (pars tensa)

Important elements in the assessment of this patient

 • Duration of ear symptoms, associated infective episodes, current otalgia or discharge, imbalance or vertigo (at presentation or previously), tinnitus, patient's perception of hearing
- Childhood hearing concerns or pathology? Childhood grommets/history of Eustachian tube dysfunction
- Previous ear surgery?
- Status of, and symptoms in, contralateral/better hearing ear
- Sinonasal symptoms and disease
- Water exposure
- Impact on life and work (always establish occupation); concerns and expectations of the patient
- Examination: Otoscopy, facial nerve, tuning fork tests. Always assess the other ear!

Management of disease

You should stress that this is primarily a surgically treated disease and the approach you would take is in line with your training. Your emphasis should be on counselling the patient on the natural history of a middle ear cholesteatoma, and the benefits and relative risks of surgical intervention. These include outlining the complications of the disease process and presenting the primary goals of the procedure. That is to achieve a safe, dry ear, and with a secondary aim of hearing improvement. In an elderly patient with significant comorbidities, or in an only-hearing ear, there remains a role for conservative management. In such a situation, with potential risks of such a management strategy, you may wish to emphasise that you would seek a second opinion.

What are the complications of untreated cholesteatoma?

The complications of untreated cholesteatomas are worth knowing in detail. They can be broadly classified as extracranial and intracranial.

The most common complications are as follows:

- Extracranial: subperiosteal abscess, Bezold abscess, zygomatic abscess, lateral semicircular canal fistula, ossicular erosion, facial nerve palsy
- Intracranial: meningitis, lateral sinus thrombosis, cerebral abscess.

In the context of either chronic otitis media or cholesteatoma, the quoted risk for intracranial complications is 1/3500.

What investigations would you arrange?

Pure tone audiogram: What are the hearing thresholds, and have they remained stable? What are the thresholds in the better hearing ear?

Beware of interpreting an audiogram in bilateral maximal conductive hearing loss, when it may not be feasible to mask, and therefore not possible to determine which ear the bone conduction relates to.

Imaging: Imaging is mandatory for anyone in training now and in the near future it will become an absolute requirement. Demonstrate that imaging may support your management approach including supporting a diagnosis (scutum and ossicular erosion), assessing for complications and therefore counselling of the patient pre-operatively (erosion of the lateral semi-circular canal [LSCC] – significantly increased risk of a dead ear, relationship to, or bony dehiscence over the facial nerve), assessing of suitability for CWU surgery (tegmen height, jugular bulb – location and dominance, pneumatisation of mastoid), or defining the extent of disease. Ensure that your approach to imaging is in line with a robust approach to managing and treating cholesteatoma.

CT: Good bony anatomy, used to demonstrate evidence of ossicular or bone erosion

MRI: (diffusion weighted, non-echo planar imaging 'non-EPI dwMRI') plays a role in defining the extent of disease and informing surgical planning; more useful in recurrent cholesteatoma, a chronically discharging perforation or after blind sac closure.

The debatable areas which you should be able to discuss

The approach is dependent on the disease process and its extent, patient factors and an individual's training in ear surgery (exposure to CWU, CWD, endoscopic, mastoid obliteration techniques).

What you offer should depend on your direct experience and you should present a plan based on your current practice, in line with an accepted approach. This might require you to acknowledge that there are alternative approaches to both working up the patient with imaging and undertaking mastoid surgery.

Canal-wall-up versus Canal-wall-down

The well-worn otology debate between a CWU and CWD approach remains relevant, but now added to the mix is the question of whether performing a mastoid obliteration or adopting a pure or combined endoscopic approach further improves recurrence rates or hearing outcomes.

Be prepared to offer the positives and negatives of a CWU versus CWD approach (see Heywood RL and Narula AA. *Otorhinolaryngologist* 2013;6(3):140–14), and the place of back-to-front (CWU) or front-to-back (CWD) approaches to the disease.

A CWU approach, otherwise known as a combined approach tympanoplasty, provides an opportunity for a normal, self-cleaning canal that would better accommodate a hearing aid allowing continued water exposure and aquatic activities. There are higher rates of recidivism (residual or recurrent disease), though these may be reduced by performing an obliteration of the attic/mastoid. If the patient is likely to fail to attend follow up, or if frail and comorbid conditions influence suitability for multiple procedures, a CWD 'open cavity' approach may be preferable.

Recidivism is higher for CWU approaches when compared with CWD approaches in adults. Despite this, you should acknowledge there may still be reasonable rates of revision for CWD techniques. An open cavity technique forms a mastoid cavity that is likely to require periodic microscopic dewaxing, water entry causing infections and problems fitting a hearing aid, as well as cosmetic issues with a large meatoplasty. A CWD procedure is more likely than CWU to continue to experience a 'wet ear' following surgery (17% vs 10%). Mastoid obliteration techniques can also be applied to the CWD 'front-to-back' approach.

Hearing reconstruction can be performed at the primary procedure, and in a CWU approach this may be preferable as follow up may involve imaging rather than second-look procedures. Probability of hearing improvement is greater in a CWU than CWD technique (30% vs. 12% from the UK National Comparative audit). A type 3 tympanoplasty in an open cavity may still achieve reasonable hearing outcomes, and ossiculoplasty outcomes remain difficult to predict. If commenting on hearing, be able to apply the Glasgow Benefit Plot or Belfast Rule of Thumb.

Mastoid obliteration techniques

Including autologous bone or cartilage, hydroxyapatite granules.

Endoscopic techniques

Whilst these may allow purely permeatal approaches, the same principles of cholesteatoma surgery exist, namely to create a dry, safe ear.

Facial nerve monitoring

'*I would perform surgery routinely using a facial nerve monitor*'.

A facial nerve monitor is considered standard of care. You should know what the monitor offers and how it is set up: e.g. 2-channel, 4-channel; stimulator; levels of stimulation that would be expected (5 mA in bone, <2 mA directly). Requires a current stimulator, EMG electrodes, amplifier and speaker.

Consider what you might do in the event of a recognised facial nerve injury, either during mastoid surgery, or in the event of an immediate or delayed, partial or complete palsy. Have an understanding of the role of ENG and EMG testing of a facial nerve palsy in the post-operative setting.

For an excellent summary of the operative approach to identifying the facial nerve in the temporal bone [though in the context of facial nerve decompression surgery], visit https:// www.jlo.co.uk/video/facial-nerve-decompression/

Why is there a persistent discharging cavity following CWD surgery?

- Recidivism
- Narrow meatoplasty
- Excess bone over the facial nerve at the entry to the cavity (so-called 'high facial ridge')
- Cavity factors – inadequate saucerisation with remnant air cells; a relative sump
- Perforation of the neotympanum

Monitoring for recidivism

Summarise the role of MRI: Have a basic understanding of non-EPI (EPI) dW imaging. Be aware that previous MRI techniques (delayed contrast MRI, EPI dwMRI) offered less sensitivity; Non-EPI dwMRI is a highly specific technique for monitoring and for recidivism and allows detection of a >2 mm cholesteatoma.

Be aware that there is a reducing role of second-look surgery in CWU surgery, particularly with increasing acceptability of dwMRI, but that the published data means dwMRI hasn't yet been universally accepted. The second-look procedure offers a chance to perform ossicular reconstruction if not undertaken primarily.

Other considerations:

- Role for a blind sac closure: This may be considered following a revision of a cavity, and intensive medical management with poor residual hearing. It will create a maximal conductive hearing loss and alternative hearing rehabilitation options need to be considered (BCHIs).
- The impact of surgery in children: Cholesteatoma is considered to be a more aggressive disease. Greater consideration should be given to the quality of life impact of CWD surgery and potential benefits of obliteration and endoscopic techniques.
- Cholesteatoma in the only-hearing ear: Surgical versus ongoing medical management.
- Appreciate the merits of a single stage CWD approach versus leaving disease over any apparent dehiscent LSCC or cochlea. You should be able to discuss how to manage a LSCC fistula identified intraoperatively – tackled last in the dissection and bone paté used to close defect, vs. an open cavity technique and the cholesteatoma matrix left in place, mandating long-term follow up and care when microsuctioning.
- Petrous apex cholesteatoma: Appearances on CT and MRI including value of non-EPI DWI scan.
- Use of KTP laser in cholesteatoma management and its role in reducing recurrence.

Chronic Otitis Media

JOSEPH MANJALY

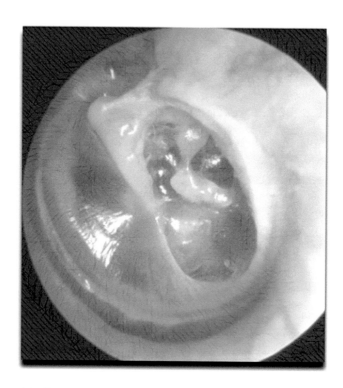

In your early training years, you may have looked at this photograph with the main aim of excluding cholesteatoma and deciding if the retraction is stable. In reality there is so much more that needs to be assessed and you need to be able to deliver those thoughts concisely and comprehensively to avoid being taken down a difficult path by the examiner. Would you operate on this ear? Would you request any imaging? There isn't necessarily always one correct answer but you need to be clear about the reasons for your answers for each case.

Could you describe what you see here?

'*This is an otoendoscopic image of a left TM, demonstrating a clean posterior pars tensa retraction, through which can be seen the stapes head in discontinuity with an eroded incus long process. On the Sade classification, this would represent a grade 3 or 4 depending on the ability to elevate the pocket with the Valsalva manoeuvre. The appearances are consistent with chronic otitis media likely secondary to poor Eustachian tube function*'.

In a chronic pars tensa retraction, the long process of incus (LPI) is usually the first to erode due to its relatively poor blood supply. Correlate this with the patient's audiogram which would be expected to show a conductive hearing loss.

Other key areas in your assessment

- Hearing loss: Duration and rate of progression will be important in counselling patients around conservative versus surgical intervention.
- Discharge and the need for repeat microsuction: Would a further endoscopic examination help visualise round corners and exclude cholesteatoma?
- Does the TM reinflate on Valsalva? One that reinflates will arguably be easier to reinforce surgically, though could also be considered a positive prognostic indicator towards resolution.
- Consider the other ear: Is it retracted? Can you infer anything about the current and previous quality of middle ear ventilation and its impact on your management? Examine the post-nasal space. Is hearing reduced contralaterally? Remember the Belfast rule of thumb and Glasgow benefit plot and their suggested relevance to ossiculoplasty.

Refer to the chapter on ossiculoplasty. Be able to explain Sade and Tos classifications of pars tensa and flaccida retractions.

What is the role of CT scanning in chronic ear disease?

There is no evidence of cholesteatoma in this photograph and you may reasonably suggest that the radiation of a CT scan is not warranted in this scenario since it will not change your management. Be clear in your mind what a CT *is* useful for though:

- Degree of mastoid pneumatisation
- Sigmoid sinus position
- Jugular bulb position
- Tegmen position
- Indicating the possible extent of disease – beware of false positives/false reassurance
- Facial nerve dehiscence
- Ossicular status
- Semicircular canal dehiscence/fistula

What are the management options in this case?

Consider carefully the aims of surgery and the patient's wishes and be able to clearly justify your reasoning.

A grommet or T-tube may be considered to try and re-ventilate the middle ear. This can be particularly useful in children where a marked reversal in retraction is sometimes seen. Beyond this, surgical intervention can be undertaken in the form of a cartilage tympanoplasty, lifting out the retraction and placing (usually tragal) cartilage underneath to prevent progression and re-retraction. This option also allows for hearing restoration with ossiculoplasty.

Most commonly used techniques are bone cement to reattach a shortened LPI back to the stapes head, or titanium prostheses: A PORP linking cartilage to the stapes head or a TORP linking cartilage to the stapes footplate. Some surgeons use the more traditional method of refashioning and replacing the existing ossicles.

 Be aware of the Wullstein classification of tympanoplasty, as well as the 2017 IOOG classification of tympanomastoid surgery: SAMEO-ATO.

You should be ready for the counter arguments to surgical intervention. Safely lifting the entire TM may be technically difficult in the most adherent middle ear. Concerns may exist around trauma to the ossicles and inner ear, and also the possibility of trapping squamous tissue under your graft. The underlying problem of Eustachian tube dysfunction is not solved by this solution. Some may argue that the hearing can be rehabilitated in other ways. Conservative management may include water precautions, hearing aid use, education and repeated microsuction. Other considerations include repeated Valsalva, Otovent, nasal steroids (though there is no good evidence for OME alone) and any role for a hearing aid or a bone conduction device. Ultimately, understand all the options well and be sure to say what *you* would do.

Cochlear Implantation

ROBERT NASH AND JOSEPH MANJALY

A 60-year-old man presents to your clinic with a history of gradual hearing loss. Please describe this audiogram.

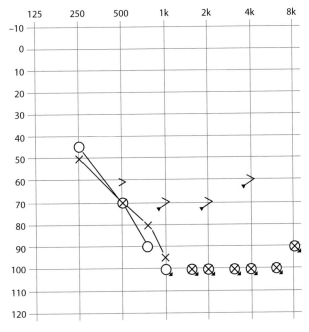

'*This is a pure tone audiogram showing bilateral moderate to profound sensorineural hearing loss. A mixed component cannot be excluded as bone conduction vibrotactile thresholds have been reached*'.

It is important to be very familiar with audiograms, even symbols that are not used commonly in ENT practice, like aided threshold levels, maximum comfortable levels, masking thresholds reached and so on. A knowledge of the rules of masking is also essential for both parts of the exam.

Important elements in the history

- Age of the patient
- Degree to which symptoms are affecting patient: Functional hearing, situations where hearing is a problem for example communication issues at home or at work
- Other symptoms: Otorrhoea, otalgia, tinnitus, vertigo
- History of hearing loss: Side, timeframe, hearing aid use (as an indicator of cortical stimulation)
- Past medical history: Including ototoxic drug exposure, previous ear surgery

How would you manage this patient?

There are more points to be scored than 'referral for hearing aids'. Mentioning types of hearing aids that may be appropriate, and how hearing aids are fitted is desirable. A basic knowledge of the types of aid (for example BTE, moulded) is useful for both parts of the examination. You may also consider behavioural interventions – tell the patient to maintain eye contact to facilitate lip reading, ask people to repeat themselves if they can't hear and so on.

Are there any other interventions that may be beneficial?

'This patient may be a candidate for cochlear implantation. NICE guidelines recommend consideration of cochlear implantation for people with thresholds of an average of >80 dB in both ears at 2 frequencies between 0.5–4 kHz who receive inadequate benefit from their hearing aids. For adults, adequate benefit is defined as a phoneme score of 50% or greater on the Arthur Boothroyd word test presented at 70 dBA. For children, adequate benefit is defined as speech, language and listening skills appropriate to age, developmental stage and cognitive ability. If criteria were met, candidacy would involve assessment by a MDT and further investigations including CT/MRI scanning'.

How does a cochlear implant work?

'Cochlear implants use externally worn speech processors to detect sound and encode it in a digital format. These appear similar to hearing aids and can be removed when the device is not in use. When in use, the signal is then communicated via two antennae held in proximity to one another by an internal and external magnet to an internally implanted receiver-stimulator package. This package then passes electrical pulses through an electrode that is implanted within the cochlea. This electrical signal directly stimulates the neurons in the spiral ganglion, providing the sensation of sound via existing auditory pathways'.

What factors are important when considering which side to implant?

Currently, in contrast to children who are offered bilateral surgery, the NHS only provides unilateral cochlear implantation to adult patients within criteria who do not have an additional sensory impairment. The MDT assessment needs to consider the following issues when choosing which side to implant:

- How much residual hearing is there? It may be preferable to implant the worse ear and preserve acoustic hearing in the better hearing ear.
- Which is the 'better connected' ear? A careful history should be taken to ascertain how much sound input the brain has received through each ear over the course of the patient's life. This means asking about the cause, time course and progression of the patient's hearing loss, and the history of hearing aid use in each ear. Implanting an ear that has been profoundly deaf and unaided for many years is likely to yield poorer outcomes compared to a well stimulated ear where the hearing has recently dropped.
- Are there any anatomical issues on cross-sectional imaging? Cochlear morphology and the presence of a vestibulocochlear nerve should be evaluated.
- Are there any functional anatomical issues? E.g. a patient with a shoulder problem who can't lift one of their arms to adjust their processor.
- Does the patient have any balance difficulties? Consider vestibular hypofunction and the consequences of the patient losing any residual balance function.
- Does the patient have a preference?

How is a cochlear implant inserted?

Cochlear implant surgery is performed on appropriately assessed and consented patients. A facial nerve monitor must be used. A post-auricular incision is made, a cortical mastoidectomy and posterior tympanotomy are drilled, and the round window niche is exposed. In some implants, a bed is fashioned below temporalis, and the implant package is placed in this bed. The round window membrane is opened or alternatively a cochleostomy is drilled, and the implant is inserted into the cochlea slowly to maximise the chance of preserving any residual acoustic hearing. Electrophysiological testing may be undertaken at the time of surgery or at a later date.

 NICE: Cochlear implants for children and adults with severe to profound deafness, available at https://www.nice.org.uk/guidance/ta566

Ear drops and Anaesthetics

JOSEPH MANJALY

Here's a handy table of agents you commonly use, just in case you get asked what's in them!

Name	Contents
Sofradex	Framycetin, Gramicidin and Dexamethasone
Gentisone HC	Gentamicin 0.3% + Hydrocortisone 1%
Otosporin	Hydrocortisone +Neomycin+ Polymixin B
Otomize	Dexamethasone + Neomycin + Acetic acid
Locorten-Vioform	Flumetasone Pivalate + Clioquinol
Betnesol-N	Betamethasone + Neomycin
Canestan	Clotrimazole 1% Don't use with perforation
Triadcortyl ointment	Triamcinolone, Neomycin, Gramicidin, Nystatin
Lignospan	2% lidocaine (20mg/ml) + 1:80,000 adrenaline. 2.2ml cartridge = 44mg Lidocaine
Co-phenylcaine	5% Lidocaine + 0.5% Phenylephrine

Be aware of the ENT UK guidelines on the use of aminoglycoside topical antibiotics in the presence of a TM perforation.

Essentially, try to use an alternative first, and if you have to use them, do so for no longer than 2 weeks and explain the rationale and risks to the patient. It may be worth asking about family history, given that the m.1555A>G variant confers susceptibility to aminoglycoside-mediated hearing loss.

Facial Palsy

NISHCHAY MEHTA

Tell me the course of the facial nerve

The facial nerve controls the muscles of facial expression, conveys taste sensation from the anterior two thirds of the tongue and supplies preganglionic parasympathyetic fibres to head and neck ganglia. The course of the facial nerve can be split into intracranial, intra-temporal and extra-temporal parts. The intra-temporal part of the facial nerve can be further divided into meatal, labyrinthine, tympanic and mastoid segments.

The meatal segment of the facial nerve is covered in meninges and accounts for the facial nerve from the porous acousticus to the fundus (13–15 mm).

The labyrinthine segment is the narrowest (0.7 mm) and accounts for the facial nerve from the fundus of the IAM to the geniculate ganglion (4 mm).

The tympanic segment (8–11 mm) accounts for the facial nerve between the first and second genu (marked by the pyramidal eminence). It courses on the medial wall of the middle ear deep to cochleariform process and over the top of the oval window to the pyramidal eminence. It has no branches within this section.

The mastoid segment accounts for the nerve from the second genu to the stylomastoid foramen (10–14 mm).

The extratemporal facial nerve extends from the stylomastoid to the pes anserinus (15–20 mm).

 Watching online animated videos of the course of the facial nerve can be a helpful way of learning this.

Do you know of any classification system for nerve-related trauma?

 Sunderland's classification of nerve trauma:

- Class I: Neuropraxia where there is a temporary conduction block without interrupting the endo-, peri- or epineurium.
- Class 2: Axonotmesis, which is a disruption of the axon but not the endo-, peri- or epineurium.
- Class 3: Damage to axon and endoneurium but not the perineurium or epineurium.
- Class 4: Damage to all layers apart from epineurium
- Class 5: Complete transection.

The endoneurium is a tightly adherent layer that surrounds each axon. The perineurium surrounds multiple endoneural tubules and provides tensile strength and protection from infections. The epineurium is the outermost layer and contains the vasa nervorum.

Recovery from Class I is complete but may take weeks. In Class 2, Wallerian degeneration occurs distal to site of injury but axonal regeneration within the connective tissue framework leads to recovery without intervention within months. Recovery from Class 3 damage is possible but rarely complete or without dysfunction (e.g. synkinesis). Both Classes 4 and 5 would require surgical intervention.

 Be aware of Seddon's three-level classification system as well which may be more appropriate to inflammatory causes of facial paralysis. Class 1: neuropraxia, Class 2: axonotmesis, Class 3: neurotmesis.

Do you know of any grading classification systems of facial palsy?

'The most commonly used classification system for facial paralysis includes the House–Brackmann 6-point scale with 1 representing normal, 2 barely perceptible weakness, 3 obvious weakness, but complete eye closure, 4 incomplete eye closure but symmetry at rest, 5 barely perceptible movement and asymmetry at rest and 6 no movement at all'.

The House–Brackmann 6-point scale fails to describe synkinesis, muscle contractures or allow classification of different muscle groups. Additionally, it has considerable inter-rater variability and has a limited role in predicting prognosis. The Sunnybrook scale is a newer classification system that has addressed some of these issues but because of increased complexity has failed to overtake House–Brackmann in popularity. Prognosis can occasionally be predicted by electrophysiological tests.

Electroneuronograph (ENoG) tests electrical propagation along the facial nerve from the stylomastoid foramen to facial muscles and compares it to the normal contralateral side. If an injury is proximal to the stylomastoid foramen then Wallerian degeneration will take 72 hours to travel from the injured site (usually ear) to the stylomastoid foramen. Therefore, ENoG done within 72 hours of onset of facial paralysis will provide a false positive result as the segment of facial nerve from the stylomastoid foramen to facial muscles is completely unaffected. Additionally, Wallerian degeneration is complete from the site of injury to muscles at 21 days, at which point all excitability is lost along the nerve. The severity of the injury cannot be assessed beyond this time frame as all injuries above Class I will show a negative result. A 10% response at day 10 of facial palsy is highly correlated to incomplete recovery. ENoG can thus be considered in patients with complete facial paralysis between days 3 and 21 post onset, to assess prognosis and further management.

What are the common causes of facial nerve palsy?

More than half of peripheral facial nerve palsies are idiopathic and termed Bell's palsy. The most commonly cited theory for aetiology of Bell's palsy is reactivation of HSV-1 in the geniculate ganglion.

Facial nerve palsy can be central or peripheral. The most common cause of central facial paralysis is a stroke. Central causes result in forehead sparing due to bilateral cortical representation of the frontalis muscle.

Peripheral nerve palsies can be divided into congenital and acquired. Congenital palsies include Möbius syndrome where there is bilateral facial weakness associated with limb abnormalities including club foot, strabismus and a weak tongue. Acquired facial palsies can be secondary to infections such as reactivation of latent varicella zoster virus in the geniculate ganglion giving painful vesicles in the conchal bowl of the pinna, acute otitis media and necrotising otitis externa, trauma (penetrating to the face or blunt causing temporal bone fractures) and iatrogenic (commonly tympanic and mastoid segments of facial nerve), tumours such as vestibular and facial schwanommas, and inflammatory conditions such as Melkersson-Rosenthal syndrome.

Acute otitis media causes facial palsy through infection affecting a dehiscent facial nerve.

Necrotising otitis externa (NOE) causes facial palsy by compression of the stylomastoid segment. Facial schwanommas are benign and are only considered for treatment if the House–Brackmann score is 4 or more, since treatments rarely give House–Brackmann scores better than 3. Melkersson-Rosenthal syndrome is an inflammatory condition that presents with recurring facial swellings and fissured tongues.

What is the prognosis of Bell's palsy?

'*85% start to see improvement within 3 weeks, 85% return to normal function by 9 months, 5% are left with a House–Brackmann 4 or worse*'.

What treatment would you give to a patient with Bell's palsy?

'*Once the diagnosis of Bell's palsy is made, I would initiate oral steroid treatment as well as eye protection and regular facial muscle exercises*'.

> Since most patients make a complete recovery, the aims of treatment are to prevent complications of temporary facial palsy and to increase the proportion of those who make it to complete recovery. Exposure keratitis and corneal ulcers are risk factors for untreated facial palsy, so the eye is protected using drops in the day and ointment/eye taping at night. Regular muscle exercises prevent synkinesis and speed up recovery. Large randomised controlled studies have shown benefit of early use oral steroids in patients with Bell's palsy, improving complete resolution to 93% at 9 months. There is limited evidence to support the use of antivirals.

Are there surgical options available for facial palsy?

Surgical intervention is undertaken most commonly for trauma, iatrogenic or tumour-related causes of facial paralysis. Surgical procedures can be related to the nerve or the muscle group.

Surgery to the nerve is indicated in nerve transection. It is also considered in the non-transected nerve when there is failure to recover facial function beyond House–Brackmann grade 4 at a year. Surgery in this case should ideally take place within 18 months before there is loss of muscle end plates. Techniques include end-to-end anastomoses, cable graft anastomoses, or cross facial anastomoses.

If there is healthy nerve proximal and distal to the lesion then reconnecting the two ends provides best outcomes, this can be done end to end if tension-free apposition is possible or using a cable graft such as the greater auricular. If there is healthy nerve distally but not proximally (e.g. CPA tumour) then nerve transposition techniques can be used. If the lesion causing the facial paralysis has also affected other ipsilateral CN (e.g. stroke/brain stem lesions) then one could consider cross-over transposition using facial nerve branches from the contralateral side. Alternatively, if there is the possibility of contralateral facial nerve palsy (e.g. neurofibromatosis type 2) then one would consider using an ipsilateral hypoglossal nerve transposition.

Surgery to the facial musculature can be undertaken as an adjunct to nerve surgery or when there has been sufficient wasting of facial muscles to prevent benefit from reinnervation.

Static procedures include facial slings that use synthetic material to support orbicularis oris and provide oral competence and better resting symmetry of the lower face, or brow lifts to remove ptotic brow from obscuring vision and provide symmetry to the upper face. Additionally, an upper eyelid weight implant can help with eye closure. Dynamic procedures like temporalis tendon transfer allow dynamic lip movement. Temporalis is a muscle of mastication and is thus already activated during chewing, which provides support for oral incompetence. Finally, Botox injections can be provided to reduce ipsilateral synkinesis or contralateral hypertonia.

With such a variation in cause, degree of severity and time course of symptoms in facial palsy, this can be a tricky exam topic – made harder by the fact that management strategies vary quite considerably between centres and between different countries. Even trying to describe the practice in your unit is difficult because the total numbers of each cause of non-resolving facial palsy are small in each hospital. Your best strategy will be to equip yourself with a management strategy that you can make sense of and that has an evidence base that you can justify it with.

 Here are some helpful papers:

Sun DQ, Andresen NS, Gantz BJ. Surgical management of acute facial palsy. *Otolaryngol Clin North Am.* 2018;51:1077–92.

Hohman MH, Hadlock TA. Etiology, diagnosis, and management of facial palsy: 2000 patients at a facial nerve center. *Laryngoscope.* 2014;124:E283–93.

Hohman MH, Bhama PK, Hadlock TA. Epidemiology of iatrogenic facial nerve injury: A decade of experience. *Laryngoscope.* 2014;124:260–5.

Ménière's disease

KIRAN JUMANI AND PETER KULLAR

A 50-year-old woman presents with recurrent episodes of vertigo and a sense of fullness in her left ear. She has noticed her hearing is worse on the left and at night she can hear an annoying rumbling sound in this ear.

Important elements in the history

- Episodic vertigo (tend to cluster in groups) typically 20 minutes to 4 hours but no longer than 24 hours
- Vertigo can be associated with nausea, vomiting and occasionally diarrhoea
- Fluctuating hearing: It may worsen before vertigo spells
- Fluctuating tinnitus in affected ear: It may worsen before vertigo spells
- Aural fullness (may increase prior to attack)
- Drop attacks (uncommon and tend to occur in late stages – sudden loss of balance without loss of consciousness)
- Family history/recent viral illness/autoimmune disorders are possible risk factors
  - Ask about driving
  - Ask for an audiogram

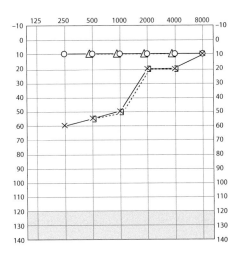

'This pure tone audiogram shows a sensorineural low frequency moderate hearing loss affecting her left ear and a normal hearing in the right ear. With the given history, the likely diagnosis is left-sided endolymphatic hydrops, probably Ménière's disease'.

In a Ménière's viva, as in clinical practice, the history is key. The clinical examination will often be unremarkable but explain you will perform a complete neurotological examination including CN 3–12 and eye movements for nystagmus, saccades and smooth pursuit. It is possible you may find evidence of peripheral vestibulopathy with a positive head-thrust test and rotation on the Unterberger stepping test.

 You could be asked to draw a diagram of the organ of Corti, give an overview of cochlear physiology and explain the pathophysiology of Ménière's disease.

Differential diagnoses for Ménière's disease

- Vestibular schwannoma
- Vestibular migraine (migraine-associated vertigo)
- Vestibular neuronitis
- Viral labyrinthitis
- BPPV
- Vertebrobasilar insufficiency
- Multiple sclerosis (MS)

Ménière's disease and its variants

'Ménière's disease is an idiopathic endolymphatic hydrops characterised by a triad of spontaneous episodic vertigo, hearing loss and tinnitus. These patients also experience aural fullness in the affected ear'.

The term 'Ménière syndrome' is used when these symptoms are secondary to a known inner ear disorder e.g. autoimmune disease or trauma.

Ménière's disease usually affects one ear, but both ears are involved in 30% of patients. In Lermoyez's variant of Ménière's disease, hearing loss and tinnitus may precede the first attack of vertigo by months or years, and the hearing may improve with onset of the vertigo.

Criteria for diagnosis of Ménière's disease and classification

The 1995 American Academy of Otolaryngology Head and Neck Foundation (AAO-HNSF) criteria of certain, definite, probable and possible Ménière's disease were amended in 2015 by the AAO-HNSF Equilibrium Committee. The classification has been simplified to:

- *Definite Ménière's disease*:
  - Two or more spontaneous episodes of vertigo, each lasting 20 min to 12 h.
  - Audiometrically documented low- to mid-frequency sensorineural hearing loss in one ear, defining the affected ear on at least one occasion before, during, or after one of the episodes of vertigo
  - Fluctuating aural symptoms (hearing, tinnitus, or fullness) in the affected ear
  - Not better accounted for by another vestibular diagnosis
- *Probable Ménière's disease*:
  - Two or more episodes of vertigo or dizziness, each lasting 20 min to 24 h

○ Fluctuating aural symptoms (hearing, tinnitus, or fullness) in the affected ear

○ Not better accounted for by another vestibular diagnosis

 Goebel JA. 2015 Equilibrium Committee Amendment to the 1995 AAO-HNS Guidelines for the Definition of Ménière's Disease. *Otolaryngol Head Neck Surg.* 2016;154(3):403–4.

What investigations would you undertake?

Pure tone audiometry is the most useful diagnostic test. An MRI scan of the head and internal auditory meati (IAM) is standard practice to rule out a lesion of the IAM/CPA or a white matter lesion e.g. MS. Increasingly, MRI with IV gadolinium is being used to look for objective evidence of hydrops. Vestibular assessment including calorics may also be useful to establish the degree of existing peripheral vestibulopathy and help guide further management. Electrocochleography (ECochG) can be performed but is primarily a research tool. A delayed cVEMP response may also be found.

How would you manage this condition?

Divide the treatment plan between vertigo, hearing, tinnitus and generalised imbalance. Ascertain which symptoms are most troublesome for the patient. Recognise there is a treatment ladder, starting from symptomatic to destructive medical and surgical procedures. Appropriate treatment will be individualised to the patient depending on the severity of their symptoms.

Symptomatic medical treatments

- *Vestibular suppressants*: Used in symptomatic vertigo attacks (e.g. prochlorperazine, cinnarizine). Overuse impairs compensation and contributes to decompensation. Sublingual options are also available e.g. Buccastem
- *Vestibular rehabilitation*: For generalised imbalance
- *Hearing aids and hearing therapy*: Rehabilitate hearing and tinnitus retraining therapy
- Psychological support for commonly associated problems of anxiety and depression

Lifestyle, alcohol, caffeine and salt restriction (both alcohol and caffeine can result in vasoconstriction and reduction in blood supply to the inner ear; salt restriction can control both volume and composition of endolymph).

 Luxford E, Berliner KI, Lee J, Luxford WM. Dietary modification as adjunct treatment in Ménière's disease: patient willingness and ability to comply. *Otol Neurotol.* 2013 Oct;34(8):1438–43.

Prophylactic treatments

- Thiazide diuretics to generally decrease the amount of fluid retention. Currently there are no drugs that specifically decrease fluid retention in the inner ear.

There is currently insufficient evidence for or against the use of diuretics in Ménière's disease.

- *Betahistine*: A histamine H3 receptor antagonist and weak H1 agonist. Postulated to work by reducing endolymphatic hydrops through improvements in microcirculation. The drug is generally well tolerated and is effective in some patients however the BEMED trial found no difference in symptom control between betahistine and placebo groups.

Adrion C, Fischer CS, Wagner J, Gürkov R, Mansmann U, Strupp M. Efficacy and safety of betahistine treatment in patients with Meniere's disease: Primary results of long-term, multicentre, double blind, randomised, placebo controlled, dose defining trial (BEMED trial). *Br Med J.* 2016;352:h6816.

Hearing preservation treatment options

- *IT steroid injections*: Methylprednisolone/dexamethasone – these work just as well as IT gentamicin and cause less morbidity e.g. worsening hearing levels.

Patel M, Agarwal K, Arshad Q et al. IT methylprednisolone versus gentamicin in patients with unilateral Ménière's disease: A randomised, double blind, comparative effectiveness trial. *Lancet* 2016;388:2753–62.

- *Saccus decompression*: Removal of bone over the saccus endolymphaticus is highly controversial and could have no more than a placebo effect. Based on theory that it alters the drainage/absorption of fluid from inner ear. Recently, clipping of the endolymphatic duct has also been described.

Sham study: Bretlau P, Thomsen J, Tos M, Johnsen NJ. Placebo effect in surgery for Meniere's disease: A three-year follow-up study of patients in a double blind placebo controlled study on endolymphatic sac shunt surgery. *Am J Otol* 1984;5:558–61). Also see surgical landmarks and Donaldson's line for endolymphatic sac.

- *Grommet insertion*: Anecdotally effective in some patients. Can be used to administer positive pressure therapy e.g. Meniett device.

Refer to 'Micropressure for refractory Meniere's disease' (NICE interventional procedure guidance 426, April 2012). Cochrane review 'Positive pressure therapy for Meniere's disease or syndrome' found no evidence supporting its use.

Ablative treatments

- Aminoglycosides: Vestibulotoxic agent acting as a partial chemolabyrinthectomy, via a mechanism involving NMDA receptor binding and production of reactive oxygen species.

Systematic reviews found 90% symptom control e.g. Huon LK, Fang TY, Wang PC. Outcomes of IT gentamicin injection to treat Ménière's disease. *Otol Neurotol* 2012;33:706–14.

- *Vestibular nerve section*: Neurosurgical/neurotological procedure considered if failed gentamicin treatment, aims to control vertigo and preserve hearing.
- *Labyrinthectomy*: Drilling out the whole of the inner ear, may be considered where there is no serviceable hearing.

Ménière's disease and the DVLA

DVLA guidance for doctors states that patients should not drive if they are liable to 'attacks of unprovoked or unprecipitated disabling giddiness'.

 Refer to DVLA. At a glance guide to the medical standards of fitness to drive: for medical practitioners. 2014.

Necrotising Otitis Externa

NISHCHAY MEHTA

Please describe the image

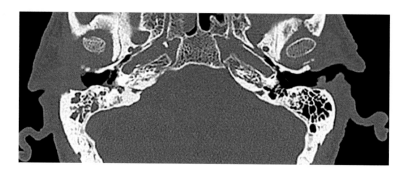

'*This is an axial cut of a CT scan at the level of the temporal bones. There is opacification of the right mastoid air cells and soft tissue filling the lateral ear canal. There is erosion of mastoid cortex laterally and erosive changes along the anterior canal wall with sequestration of bone and loss of mandibular head cortex. My differential for such a process would include necrotising otitis externa (skull base osteomyelitis), ORN, and ear canal malignancy*'.

Have a rapid method to evaluate CT scans of the temporal bone in axial and coronal planes. The cochlea, labyrinth, ossicles and facial nerve are high yield structures for surgical pathology. Each one can be evaluated in turn and so it is important to know how to initially identify them.

Findings specific to NOE include obliteration of the normal fat planes in the subtemporal area as well as patchy destruction of the bony cortex of the mastoid. The point of exit of the various CN can be identified on CT scans, and the extent of the inflammatory mass correlates well with the clinical findings. MRI with gadolinium is the best modality to assess for the soft tissue changes associated with NOE.

What is necrotising otitis externa?

'*Necrotising otitis externa is an infection of the outer ear that has spread to the bone of the skull base*'.

The fissures of Santorini are natural breaks in the hyaline cartilage of the EAC that allow infection to spread from the ear to the skull base. The foramen of Huschke is a natural dehiscence antero-inferiorly in the bony EAC (U-shaped tympanic ring) that usually persists until adolescence and allows infections and malignancy to spread between the ear and the parotid space.

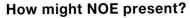

How might NOE present?

'*NOE is most common in the immunocompromised, particularly the elderly and diabetics. It usually occurs as a progression of a non-resolving otitis externa associated with severe otalgia. Discharge and inflammation are noted on microscopic examination with granulation seen at the junction of the ear canal cartilage and bone. There is often exposed bone in the canal*'.

Patients with diabetes have more alkaline wax, reduced function of white cells and end vessel vasculitis that leaves them prone to ear infections.

The infection can spread from skin of the external ear canal along the fissures of Santorini within the lateral ear cartilage to the lateral skull base. Osteomyelitis can spread anteriorly to the temporo-mandibular joint and masseter space and cause trismus or along the skull base medially and irritate the CN either through neurotoxin release or direct compression by inflammatory tissue. Medially infection spreads to the central skull base by tracking from the petrous bone to the clivus.

CN palsies occur in less than a quarter of patients but are associated with poorer outcomes. The facial nerve is the most commonly reported palsy and the stylomastoid foramen is the commonly reported site for compromise.

What is the most common pathogen involved?

'*Pseudomonas aeruginosa, a Gram-negative rod, is the most commonly cultured bacteria in NOE. It is opportunistic and only a pathogen when the host's immune system is deficient. Local invasion causes a coagulative necrosis and the bacteria additionally has the ability to produce lytic enzymes, endotoxins and neurotoxins*'.

 Pseudomonas aeruginosa, Staphylococcus aureus, Proteus mirabilis, Aspergillus flavus and *Candida* species are commonest organisms related to NOE.

How do you make the diagnosis?

'*The diagnosis is made when at-risk patients have non-resolving otitis externa associated with severe otalgia, granulation at the bony-cartilaginous ear canal junction, and raised ESR/CRP as well as positive microbiology and histology showing inflammation without neoplasia. Imaging is used to confirm diagnosis and can be used to monitor treatment*'.

A combination of pain score and CRP/ESR are the most useful markers of clinical progression (although otalgia may be minimal in severely immunocompromised patients e.g. post-transplant).

What imaging techniques would you consider for a patient with suspected NOE?

CT is a rapid and inexpensive screening test that can reveal location and extent of the disease but only demonstrates abnormality once one-third of the bone is demineralised. MRI scanning is considered the best modality to identify soft tissue changes and bone marrow oedema. Nuclear medicine scans such a Gallium-67 are infrequently used due to low specificity. It should be noted that imaging findings lag behind the clinical response to treatment.

How do you manage patients with NOE?

'*These patients are managed by an MDT including ENT, infectious diseases, microbiology and neuroradiology with endocrinology and pain teams if required. Treatment requires tight monitoring and control of blood sugars, and long-term administration of microbiological appropriate antibiotics through long lines, as well as complex pain management. Current protocols dictate a minimum of 6 weeks IV then 6 weeks oral antibiotics. I use the clinical picture, ESR and CRP to determine when to stop treatment. Repeat MRI is used if the clinical picture does not improve. Biopsies are taken at the start of treatment to exclude ear canal squamous cell carcinoma (SCC)*'.

Patients with NOE represent a particular challenge as they often have considerable pre-existing medical conditions that have got worse due to their infection. For example, in diabetics glycaemic control is often difficult to maintain, and antibiotic treatment often results in an insult to a poorly functioning renal system. Additionally, their antibiotic regime needs close monitoring, in light of antimicrobial resistance, especially if long lines are inserted and outpatient antibiotic treatment is considered.

Noise-induced Hearing Loss

JAMEEL MUZAFFAR

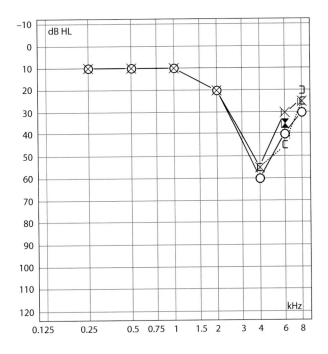

'This is a pure tone audiogram showing symmetrical sensorineural thresholds with a notch at 4 kHz bilaterally. This would be typical for NIHL'.

A typical way to begin an NIHL viva would be with an audiogram like the one shown. Talk through the history if not already given to you. History taking is similar to any other otological complaint but must pay particular attention to occupational and social noise exposure. This may include noisy machinery or working environments, listening to personal audio equipment, attending nightclubs or live music venues or hobbies such as clay pigeon shooting. It is also important to ascertain what hearing protection, if any, has been worn. The clinical examination will typically be unremarkable but should be mentioned for completeness. There may be a medico-legal aspect to the scenario so familiarity with the Control of Noise at Work (2005) legislation is helpful. If the scenario features a serving or veteran person in the Armed Forces, an awareness of significantly increased rates of hearing impairment and tinnitus amongst these groups should be mentioned.

What is NIHL?

'NIHL is damage to hearing as a result of acoustic exposure. It is typically divided into temporary (TTS) and permanent threshold shifts (PTS). A TTS is a measurable worsening of hearing thresholds following an acoustic exposure that resolves typically over a period of a few days. If the impairment does not resolve it is termed a PTS'.

Important elements in the history

 • Infections/trauma/previous surgery/ototoxic medication
  • Age of onset, progression of hearing loss
  • Family history (several genes appear to increase pre-disposition to NIHL)
  • Vertigo
  • Tinnitus
  • Ask about current and previous occupational and social noise exposure as well as hearing protection worn

What is acute acoustic trauma?

'*Sudden damage to the inner ear due to excess noise exposure, typically from explosions or gunshots. These may be present alongside conductive deficits due to rupture of the TM or fracture of the ossicles*'.

What investigations would you undertake?

Generally, investigations beyond pure tone audiometry are not indicated. If there is significant asymmetry or something else about the history seems odd, MRI is the investigation of choice (as typical for other sensorineural losses).

How would you manage this condition?

Management of chronic NIHL can be divided into hearing rehabilitation, prevention of further damage and occupational aspects.

Hearing rehabilitation, typically with conventional air conduction hearing aids, may be indicated if the patient is struggling functionally or to help with tinnitus.

Prevention of further damage is best performed by avoiding damaging exposures, though often hobby shooters are unwilling to give up. Less effectively reducing contact or modifying the environment may help. Least effective, but essential to discuss, is hearing protection with personal protective equipment such as ear defenders.

Occupational advice should include encouraging the patient to tell their employer about their hearing loss and to ensure they are compliant with health and safety legislation.

Acute acoustic trauma may benefit from treatment with corticosteroids. IT steroids are probably superior to oral administration for initial treatment and definitely superior for salvage but administration can be uncomfortable and requires appropriate equipment. Controversy exists as to whether dexamethasone or methylprednisolone is the optimum therapy. Steroid treatment is typically offered up to 2–3 weeks post injury, though as with sudden onset sensorineural hearing loss this may not be effective. Earlier administration is better, probably the earlier the better.

What are the Control of Noise at Work Regulations 2005?

These regulations were established as part of the Health and Safety at Work Act 1974 and were last updated in 2005. They set out the framework for the protection and monitoring of employees hearing health and occupational exposures.

Below an average of 80 dB and a peak sound pressure level of 135 dB no precautions are required.

Between 80 and 85 dB average exposure or a peak exposure between 135 and 137 dB employers have a duty to assess risks to workers' health and provide appropriate information and training.

Above 85 dB average exposure or 137 dB peak sound pressure is the threshold at which hearing protection and hearing zones must be provided.

An average of 87 dB and a peak sound pressure of 140 dB represent the maximum levels to which employees may be exposed.

Non-organic Hearing Loss

KIRAN JUMANI

As mentioned in other chapters, you need to be able to interpret audiograms and describe them succinctly to get the viva off to a good start. Furthermore, having the ability to spot the distinct pattern in this particular case will help a great deal in getting to the more challenging parts of the viva early.

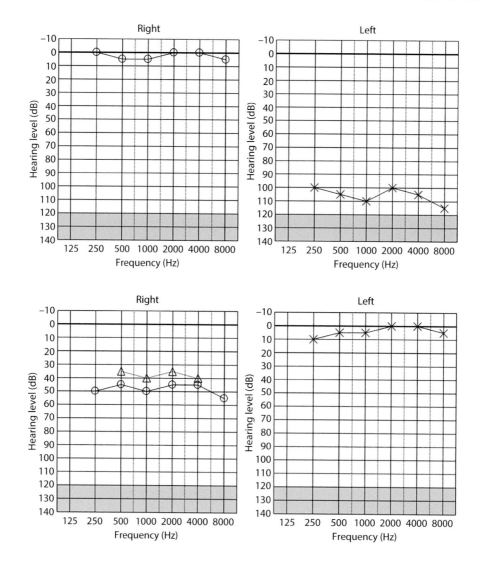

What do you think may be happening in these audiograms?

'The upper two images show an audiogram that suggests a profound almost flat hearing loss on the left side and normal hearing on the right. A large difference in unmasked thresholds greater than 40 dB between ears should raise suspicion of a spurious result. The lower two images show a moderate hearing loss on the right with unmasked bone conduction thresholds worse than the normal air conduction thresholds on the left. In this case, one would expect unmasked bone conduction thresholds on the right to match the air conduction thresholds on the left, raising suspicion of non-organic hearing loss'.

What is non-organic hearing loss?

'Non-organic hearing loss is an apparent hearing loss (or exaggeration of hearing loss) with no evidence of a physical problem to explain it. This does not include people who are unable to perform pure tone audiometry'.

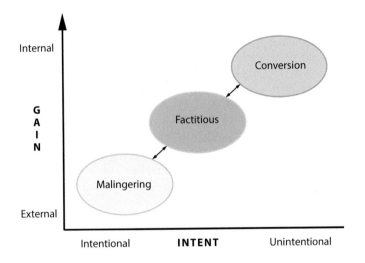

 Austen S, Lynch C. Non-organic hearing loss redefined: understanding, categorizing and managing non-organic behaviour. *Int J Audiol.* 2004;43(8):449–457.)

Malingering patients are intentional in falsifying or exaggerating symptoms. Factitious patients intentionally feign hearing loss for internal gain. Conversion patients are not intentional in responding at suprathreshold levels. By understanding the underlying motivation and degree of intent, it is easier to recognise non-organic behaviour and manage the patient appropriately. The initial strategy should be non-confrontational. If the patient has been given chances to respond appropriately yet continues to respond at suprathreshold levels (as proven by other tests), further testing to identify non-organic hearing loss should take place.

Elements of the assessment

 History

Emotional/compensation element

Examination

Conversational ability is better than the suggested by the audiogram even without lip reading

Audiogram

- Variable audiogram: Difference between ascending and descending audiometry.
- Flat tracing on audiogram: Unmasked difference between the two ears exceeding 70–80 dBHL. Stenger's test can also be performed using pure tones (Tarchanow phenomenon).

Stenger's tuning fork/audiometric test (if feigning unilateral deafness). This test is based on the auditory phenomenon known as Stenger's principle. This states that when two similar sounds are presented to both ears, only the louder of the two would be heard. When two similar tuning forks of same frequencies are made to vibrate and held simultaneously in the acoustic axis of both ears only the louder fork will be heard. Loudness of the vibrating fork can be adjusted by changing the distance of the fork from the ear canal. Usually the vibrating fork is held closer to the allegedly deaf ear of the patient. The patient will not acknowledge hearing in that ear. According to Stenger's principle he should be able to hear the louder fork. If the hearing loss in the worse ear is genuine, the patient will respond to the signal presented to the better ear. This is known as a negative Stenger's test. A patient feigning hearing loss will not acknowledge hearing the tuning fork when louder sound is presented to apparent worse ear. This is known as a positive Stenger's test.

 You may be asked to demonstrate how to perform a Stenger's test. Other tuning fork tests are Teal's test and Chimani Moos test, Erhardt's test, Lombard's test, Hummel double conversation test, delayed speech feedback test and two-tube test of Teuber.

Objective testing

- *Stapedial reflex*: If the patient denies hearing at 80 dBHL and a stapedial reflex is present at 90 dBHL this should raise suspicion. However, recruitment can cause a narrow dynamic range and abnormal loudness growth.
- *OAE*: This test tells us that the outer hair cells are functioning normally but may miss dysfunction affecting other parts of the auditory pathway.
- Speech testing better than thresholds should raise suspicion but patients can feign this test too
- *ABR*: This can be difficult to perform in adults due to myogenic interference.
- *Cortical evoked response audiometry*: A frequency-specific test, recording signals in the auditory cortex when sound is played. This is a time and labour-intensive test and typically has a role in medico-legal assessment.

Management in these patients should be tactful, objective, firm and consider an onward referral if needed.

Ossiculoplasty

NIKUL AMIN

A patient presents to your clinic with a history of hearing loss. Please describe the following audiogram.

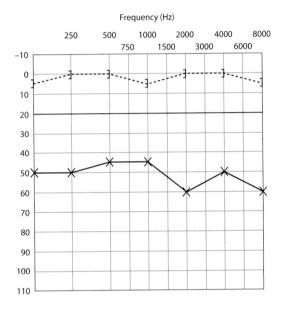

'This is a pure tone audiogram showing a left sided maximal conductive hearing loss. I would take a history and perform an examination including otoscopy to determine possible causes'.

What are the possible causes of this audiogram finding?

☑ **Outer ear disease**

- Anotia
- EAC stenosis including congential and acquired atresia
- EAC occlusion secondary to foreign bodies (although unlikely to cause a maximal conductive loss)
- Obstructive benign lesions including osteoma/exostoses
- Obstructive malignant tumours including SCC and skin cancers

Middle ear disease

- Large TM perforations
- OME

- Congenital ossicular malformation
- Discontinuity of the ossicular chain secondary to:
  - Erosive disease: Cholesteatoma, benign tumours, malignant tumours
  - Bone disease
  - Trauma
- Ossicular chain fixations including otosclerosis and tympanosclerosis

Assuming this patient has presented for a second look combined approach tympanoplasty and has no residual or recurrent cholesteatoma, what are the auditory rehabilitation options?

- Conservative measures including assistive devices and hearing therapy
- Air conduction hearing aids
- Bone conduction hearing devices
- Ossicular reconstruction
- MEI

What are the different ossicular reconstruction options?

Ossicular reconstructions can be divided broadly into PORP and TORP. Reconstruction can be performed using either autologous or synthetic materials.

 Familiarise yourself with these different types so you can recognise a picture shown to you.

When would you choose a PORP over a TORP?

This primarily depends on whether the stapes suprastructure is intact or if there is only a stapes footplate remaining. The presence of an intact stapes suprastructure appears to be an important prognostic indicator in auditory outcomes.

What options are available if the stapes footplate is absent?

A piece of cartilage can be used to replace the footplate. This is however uncommon and may worsen hearing loss. You would *not* use a TORP in this scenario.

How would you manage a patient with an isolated small incudostapedial erosion?

Options include either a PORP or reconstruction of the long and lenticular process of the incus using biocompatible bone cement.

Would you perform an ossiculoplasty as a primary procedure or at a planned second operation?

Different surgeons have different approaches to this but reasons may include concern regarding residual cholesteatoma, extensive middle ear mucosal disease, secondary ossicular disease e.g. stapes fixation.

How would you classify a successful ossiculoplasty?

A functional improvement in hearing which is often quantified as a post-operative air-bone gap ≤20 dB.

Assessing patients according to the Glasgow benefit plot can help demonstrate functional improvement post-ossiculoplasty and aid managing patients' expectations.

Understanding the Belfast rule of thumb and Glasgow Benefit Plot

The Belfast rule of thumb suggests that a patient is likely to benefit from ossicular surgery if their post-operative hearing threshold is either:

- Better than 30 dB or
- Improved to within 15 dB of the contralateral ear.

This is further appreciated when using the Glasgow benefit plot to evaluate the audiometric improvement needed for your particular patient to benefit. A point is plotted corresponding to the pre-operative thresholds for the 'ear-to-be operated' and the contralateral ear. Surgery should aim to move the patient into a new numbered group in order to confer benefit.

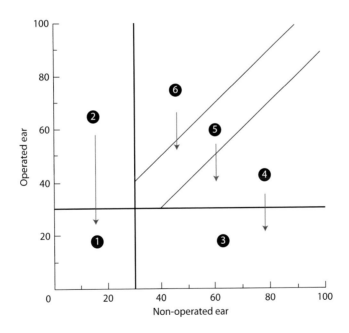

 Browning GG, Gatehouse S, Swan IR. The Glasgow Benefit Plot: A new method for reporting benefits from middle ear surgery. *Laryngoscope.* 1991;101(2):180–5.

What auditory outcomes might you expect with a PORP and a TORP?

A meta-analysis by Yu et al. in 2013 showed that PORP has significantly improved post-operative hearing outcomes along with a significantly lower rate of extrusion at long-term follow up. The use of PORP leads to a closure of the air-bone gap to less than 20 dB in over 70% of patients whilst case series using TORP between the footplate and TM noted post-operative mean ABG ≤20 dB in approximately half to two-thirds of patients.

 Yu H, He Y, Ni Y et al. PORP vs. TORP: A meta-analysis. *European Arch Oto-Rhino-Laryngol.* 2013;270:3005–17.

Poorer outcomes tend to be associated with revision surgery and ossicular chain disruption without inflammatory disease whilst improved outcomes are associated with the presence of the stapes suprastructure and malleus preservation.

What are the complications of ossiculoplasty?

Along with the routine complications related to middle ear surgery the patient may have:

- A failure to improve hearing
- Worsening hearing and complete hearing loss
- Prosthesis dislodgement. There are case reports of TORPs medialising into the vestibule resulting in hearing loss and vertigo.
- Prosthesis extrusion

Are TORP and PORP MRI safe?

There are many different materials used in TORP and PORP, however modern prostheses tend to be titanium based and the newest prostheses are conditioned for up to 7.0 T.

Otosclerosis

JOSEPH MANJALY

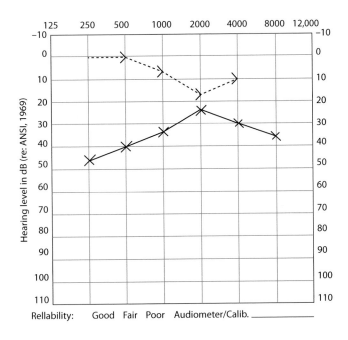

In any of the otology viva you need to be able to describe an audiogram succinctly.

'This is a pure tone audiogram showing left ear hearing thresholds of 25–45 dB. There is an air-bone gap suggestive of a conductive hearing loss, and bone conduction thresholds are 0–15 dB showing normal cochlear reserve'.

What is the significance of the dip in bone conduction at 2 kHz?

'This is an artefactual dip known as a Carhart notch, most commonly at 2 kHz, seen in conductive hearing loss which resolves upon correction of the cause (the Carhart effect). Since the natural resonance of the middle ear is 2 kHz, it may be that the middle ear contributes to normalised bone conduction measurements at this frequency'.

In an otosclerosis viva you will be typically given an audiogram like this. Talk through the history if not already given to you. The clinical examination will typically be unremarkable. Watch out for unusual patterns such as a drop in bone conduction in the high frequencies. This does not necessarily change the diagnosis or management, but it is worth showing appreciation that surgery is more likely to correct the mid- and low frequencies.

Important elements in the history

- Infections/trauma/previous surgery
- Age of onset, progression of hearing loss (in pregnancy)
- Family history
- Vertigo
- Tinnitus
- Autophony
- Occupation

Differential diagnoses for a conductive hearing loss with intact TM

- Ossicular discontinuity
- Tympanosclerosis/fixed malleus and incus
- Congenital cholesteatoma
- Paget disease
- Osteogenesis imperfecta (blue sclera)
- Note that superior semicircular canal dehiscence (SSCD) may (or may not) feature a 'pseudo conductive hearing loss' with suprathreshold bone conduction thresholds.

What is the Paracusis of Willis?

'An apparent improvement in speech perception in the presence of loud background noise, thought to be characteristic of certain types of conductive hearing loss, especially otosclerosis'.

What investigations would you undertake?

In practice this varies significantly across the country. Say what you have done in your training and be able to justify. Some consultants do none. Tuning fork tests are helpful when there is a masking dilemma and debate over which ear to treat.

Tympanometry measures TM compliance and may highlight effusion, perforation or ossicular discontinuity. Stapedial reflexes may be absent in otosclerosis. Speech discrimination testing is much more commonly used in North America. Many consultants undertake a high-resolution CT scan, which may (though not necessarily) detect otospongiosis at the *fissula ante fenestram*, and also provides information on middle ear anatomy and any alternative diagnoses.

How would you manage this condition?

Discuss a hearing aid trial and stapes surgery (undertaken with a laser or microdrill to fenestrate the stapes footplate and then place a piston attached to the incus). It is worth being able to explain in basic terms how stapes surgery is performed. The risk of a dead ear is commonly quoted as 0.5%–1% and other risks to mention include dizziness, tinnitus, altered taste, facial palsy, device failure and ear drum perforation.

What are the contraindications to surgery?

There are a number of reasons to avoid stapes surgery but there exists difference of opinion on whether any are truly strict contraindications.

Here are some of the issues you need to be aware of:

 • Infection: Avoid operating whilst actively infected
- Only-hearing ear: Can consider bone conduction devices for those unable to wear conventional aids
- Predominantly cochlear component: Is the patient within cochlear implant criteria?
- Active otosclerosis: Schwartz sign
- Glasgow benefit plot/Belfast rule of thumb: Read up on these and be able to explain/ draw the principles (see the ossiculoplasty chapter) – though remember to consider the Carhart effect in otosclerosis and the potential for the pre-operative bone conduction thresholds to be misleading.
- Occupation where dizziness/dead ear/loss of taste unacceptable
- Ménière's disease
- Aberrant facial nerve or stapedial artery (in practice this is very rare in a patient with otherwise normal morphology)

Understanding the masking dilemma and masking rules

The concept of masking can be confusing and so it is worth investing some time to understand it from first principles.

Firstly, remember that the patient needs to have a physical ear canal in order to mask air conduction. In order to 'mask' the non-test ear and prevent it detecting sound played to the test ear, one needs to play a distracting sound into the non-test ear, starting at the air conduction threshold of the non-test ear.

The volume of the masking noise is then increased by 10 dB each time the patient hears the tone until you have reached a 'plateau' – four responses to the tone without the need to increase the volume of the tone.

Now consider the problem of inter-aural attenuation. When a sound is played to one ear using standard headphones, it is assumed to be 40 dB quieter at the non-test ear. This volume difference between ears is greater when testing with insert phones where the sound is attenuated by 55 dB. For bone conduction testing we assume no attenuation at all, therefore the response is of the better hearing ear regardless of where the bone conductor was placed.

When a non-test ear has a large conductive component hearing loss, the sound needed to mask that ear may be so loud that the masking noise can be detected by the test ear. This is called the masking dilemma and means that it can be difficult to test patients with large bilateral CHLs.

There are three scenarios where masking is required that you need to know and explain (the so-called 'rules of masking'):

1. When there is an apparent ≥40 dB difference (when testing with headphones) or ≥55 dB difference (when testing with insert phones) in air conduction (AC) between the ears.

    In this scenario, mask when testing air conduction.

2. When there is an apparent >10 dB conductive loss

   In this scenario, mask the better ear when testing bone conduction at 500 Hz, 1, 2 and 4 kHz.

3. When this is an apparent ≥40 dB difference (when testing with headphones) or ≥55 dB difference (when testing with insert phones) between worse ear AC and unmasked/better bone conduction.

   In this scenario, mask the better ear when testing air conduction.

   This is similar to the Weber concept.

Acknowledgement: Thanks to Susan Eitutis, Research Audiologist at Cambridge University Hospitals, for validating the above advice.

Paraganglioma

PETER KULLAR

Please describe this image

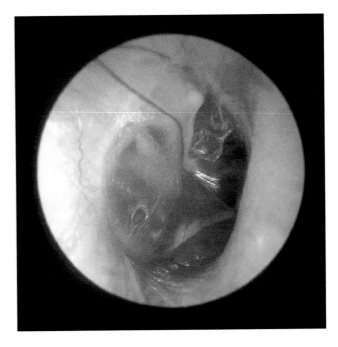

'This is an otoendoscopic image of a right TM. The most obvious abnormality is a vascular mass filling the anterior inferior quadrant. The most significant diagnosis consistent with this appearance is a jugular or tympanic paraganglioma'.

Differentials to consider

 • Haemotympanum
- Acute otitis media
- Aberrant carotid artery
- Active otosclerosis (Schwartze sign)

Paragangliomas, also less precisely called glomus tumours, are neuroendocrine tumours that arise from chemoreceptor tissue associated with the autonomic nervous system. The majority of paragangliomas are benign but malignancy can occur in around 1% of temporal bone paragangliomas and the workup in this condition is reflective of that. The blood supply of jugulotympanic paraganglioma is from the inferior tympanic branch of the ascending pharyngeal artery.

There are four types of paraganglioma that you should know about:

- Carotid body tumour
- Tympanic paraganglioma (glomus tympanicum)
- Jugular paraganglioma (glomus jugulare)
- Vagal paraganglioma (glomus vagale)

What would be the important aspects in the history and examination?

Clinical presentation is dependent on the tumour site.

Carotid body tumours typically present as a slowly enlarging, painless, lateral neck masses. As they enlarge, they will impinge on local structures causing dysphagia, CN palsies and Horner's syndrome.

Examination will reveal a non-tender neck mass at the anterior border of sternocleidomastoid that is mobile in the horizontal and not the vertical plane (Fontaine sign).

Jugular and tympanic paragangliomas present with pulsatile tinnitus and a conductive hearing loss. Otoscopic examination reveals a red/blue pulsatile retrotympanic mass (as shown).

Brown's sign is blanching of the TM on pneumatic otoscopy. Aquino sign is cessation of the pulsation of the tumour with ipsilateral compression of the carotid artery

Vagal paragangliomas present similarly but can arise from any part of the cervical vagus nerve so may additionally cause dysphonia, pain, cough, dysphagia and aspiration.

Key features in the assessment

- Age
- Conductive hearing loss, pulsatile tinnitus, neck mass
- Dysphagia and dysphonia
- CN symptoms (VII, IX-XII)
- PMH: Other tumours, chronic lung disease (hypoxia may predispose to sporadic paragangliomas)
- Family history (specifically tumour history)

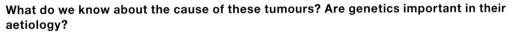

What do we know about the cause of these tumours? Are genetics important in their aetiology?

They are generally sporadic and may be associated with high altitude in some cases. In some instances, they are a feature of a syndrome including multiple endocrine neoplasia type 2 (MEN IIA and IIB caused by variants in the *RET* proto-oncogene) and von-Hippel-Lindau disease (caused by variants in the *VHL* tumour suppressor).

Hereditary paraganglioma have been shown to be associated with germline mutations in *SDHB*, *SDHC*, and *SDHD*. These genes encode subunits of mitochondrial complex II, a constituent of the electron transport chain and the citric acid cycle that plays a fundamental role in cellular respiration.

Most MDTs would undertake genetic screening in all new patients.

You suspect a jugulotympanic paraganglioma in this patient, how would you investigate further?

After a thorough history and clinical examination of the head and neck including micro-otoscopy, radiological evaluation is mandatory to establish the diagnosis.

Commonly used modalities include:

- CT (moth-eaten bony destruction)
- MRI (salt and pepper appearance) – not to be confused with salt and pepper appearance for JNAs
- Digital subtraction angiography
- Other modalities that may be considered include dynamic contrast enhanced MRA and MIBG scintigraphy
- FDG-PET is increasingly become standard to look for synchronous tumours

Awareness of these modalities shows an understanding of the complexities of the radiological investigation of head and neck paragangliomas. It is of course important to emphasise that these decisions are taken in the skull base MDT that typically includes a specialist head and neck radiologist.

As the majority of carotid and vagal paragangliomas present as lateral neck masses, the initial investigation will usually be an ultrasound scan neck±FNA. This will be supplemented by cross-sectional and nuclear medicine investigations.

Endocrine and genetics teams will carry out relevant genetic testing and plasma metanephrines will be used to rule out a synchronous phaeochromocytoma.

Can you tell me any classification systems for paragangliomas?

It is unlikely that you will be asked for the details of staging systems but it important to understand the key principles and their use in surgical decision making.

Carotid body paragangliomas

Shamblin classification: Group 1–3 (increasing difficulty of surgical resection)

Jugulotympanic paraganglioma

Fisch classification: Class A, B, C 1-4, D 1-2

Glasscock-Jackson classification: Type I–IV

Tell me about the management of paragangliomas

'Management of these tumours is based on patient factors, tumour factors and available expertise. CN function and the presence or absence of malignant features are crucial determinants'.

It is important to stress the importance of an MDT approach. Treatment is generally individualised. A period of watch and wait to determine the natural history of the tumour may be warranted particularly in patients with comorbidities, the elderly and those unwilling to undergo surgery.

Surgery is generally appropriate if there are already associated CN palsies. This may take place through the ear canal, mastoid and/or neck. It may be necessary to control the bleeding risk with pre-operative embolisation. Surgical complications include internal carotid artery injury (stroke/death) and CN palsies (risk of aspiration, tracheostomy, reliance on PEG feeding). Subtotal resection may also be considered as a way of controlling disease and preserving CN function.

Small jugular and tympanic tumours can usually be surgically excised without complication. Larger tumours necessitate the use of lateral skull base or infratemporal fossa approach. Radiotherapy can be used in patients with multiple paragangliomas and is generally well tolerated. It can be a way of avoiding CN palsies but does not relieve pulsatile tinnitus. It is associated with complications including osteroradionecrosis and the potential for secondary malignancies. For smaller tumours there is now an increasing role for stereotactic radiosurgery.

Pre-auricular Sinus

NIKUL AMIN

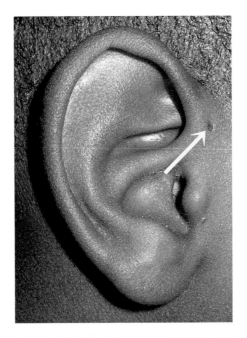

Describe this photograph

'*This is a clinical photograph of a right ear with a well-defined pit along the anterior part of the ascending helix in keeping with a pre-auricular sinus*'.

Can you explain the development of this abnormality?

Pre-auricular sinus is a congenital malformation found in approximately 1% of the population. The six hillocks of His (mesenchymal proliferations) develop the folds of the auricle from branchial arch 1 and 2 at week 6–7 gestation. Incomplete or abnormal fusion of these hillocks leads to the formation of the sinus.

Are they inherited?

They are either sporadic or inherited, especially if bilateral (approximately 20%–30% of patients). When inherited they show an autosomal dominant pattern with reduced penetrance and variable expression.

What are the symptoms?

A pre-auricular sinus is often asymptomatic with a solitary pit, most commonly just anterior to the ascending crus of the helix, although a cyst can occur. The most common presentation is recurrent infections. Whilst infected, there may be an increase in size, tenderness, surrounding erythema and discharge on palpation.

What is the differential diagnosis?

First branchial cleft anomaly (more commonly inferior and posterior to the tragus).

What conditions are associated with increased risk of a pre-auricular sinus?

Pre-auricular sinuses are also seen with increased incidence in patients with branchio-oto-renal syndrome (variant in the *EYA1* gene is identified in approximately 40% of patients). Inheritance is in an autosomal dominant pattern. Consider this diagnosis in bilateral cases and ensure audiometric testing and a renal ultrasound are carried out.

How would you treat an acute infection?

Antimicrobials – covering the common causative organisms (*Staphylococcus aureus*, *Streptococcus* spp. and *Proteus* spp.)

Admit the patient if systemically unwell, spreading facial cellulitis or failure to respond to oral antibiotics

Aspiration or incision and drainage of an abscess.

How would you treat this case?

Definitive treatment is to perform a wide local excision due to the tortuous and branching nature of the sinus tract. Dissection often involves taking a sliver of auricular cartilage and down to temporalis fascia

Definitive excision during an acute infection should be avoided for best surgical outcomes.

What is the risk of recurrence?

Performing a simple sinectomy or incomplete excision often leads to recurrence of cystic swellings and recurrent infections of up to 50%.

In cases of recurrent disease consider the use an intraoperative facial nerve monitor due to the increased fibrotic soft tissue changes distorting surgical landmarks and the potential risk of extension inferiorly towards the facial nerve.

Sensorineural Hearing Loss, Presbyacusis, Autoimmune Hearing Loss

NIKUL AMIN

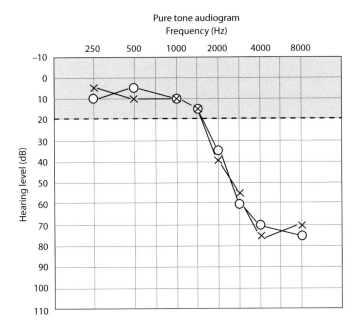

Describe the following pure tone audiogram in this 75-year-old man

'*This is a pure tone audiogram showing bilateral high frequency moderate to severe sensorineural hearing loss in keeping with possible presbyacusis*'.

What are the main different types of presbyacusis? A useful framework was proposed by Schuknecht:

- Sensory: A steep high-frequency hearing loss with preserved speech perception. Degeneration of the organ of Corti.
- Neural: Down sloping high-frequency hearing loss with a disproportionate loss of speech perception. Degeneration of spiral ganglion cells.
- Strial/metabolic: A flat sensorineural hearing loss with preserved speech perception. Degeneration of stria vascularis.
- Cochlear conductive: Progressive down sloping high-frequency sensorineural hearing loss. Increased stiffness of the basilar membrane.

Cochlear pathology in presbycusis. Schuknecht HF, Gacek MR. *Ann Otol Rhinol Laryngol.* 1993 Jan;102(1 Pt 2):1–16.

How do you diagnose presbyacusis?

'This is a clinical and audiological diagnosis of progressive hearing loss associated with aging. It presents with typically bilateral progressive symmetrical high-frequency sensorineural hearing loss with no other explanation/cause identified. Patients will often have normal examination findings on otoscopy'.

What are the broad management options?

Management is based on hearing rehabilitation using both hearing aids and hearing therapy. Bone conduction devices, MEI or cochlear implantation may be considered depending on the individual's audiometric and functional deficit.

Should all patients with presbyacusis receive hearing rehabilitation?

All patients should be appropriately counselled based on their individual requirements as failure to offer hearing rehabilitation in the elderly population has been associated with reduced quality of life, increased social isolation, depression and dementia. This is an emerging research field and good to be aware of.

Which conditions are associated with autoimmune inner ear disease?

AIED can be either ear specific or part of an established systemic autoimmune condition such as rheumatoid arthritis, Cogan syndrome, polyarteritis nodosa and SLE.

What is the cause of autoimmune hearing loss?

AIED is a rare cause of hearing loss. Self-antigen recognition by cochlear immune cells leads to activated cytotoxic lymphocytes and immunoglobulins causing immune-mediated inner ear tissue damage. Excess immune-complex deposition in the inner ear also appear to be implicated with AIED.

How would you expect a patient with suspected autoimmune hearing loss to present?

Patients may present as young as their early twenties and there is a higher prevalence in females.

Autoimmune inner ear disease presents commonly with bilateral symmetrical sensorineural hearing loss which may be rapidly progressive (weeks to months) and fluctuating.

Symptoms often start in one ear and progress to bilateral in >90% of patients.

There may be associated symptoms of imbalance, tinnitus and aural fullness in up to 50% of patients which can make it difficult to distinguish from bilateral Ménière syndrome.

What investigations should be performed?

Along with audiometry testing, laboratory investigations should be performed to attempt to identify possible antigens. This includes:

 • ESR, ANA, rheumatoid factor and antimicrosomal antibodies.

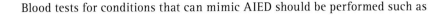

Blood tests for conditions that can mimic AIED should be performed such as

 • Syphilis, HIV and Lyme disease.

Vestibular testing (demonstrating hypofunction) and MRI scans (to rule out tumours including acoustic neuromas) can help aid the diagnosis.

How does treatment differ to other causes of sensorineural hearing loss?

Upon establishing the diagnosis the patient should receive treatment guided by the rheumatologists including oral prednisolone (1 mg/kg up to 60 mg/day).

Patients who respond can have the dose tapered although long-term treatment is often required.

Long-term IT steroid injections have been described in addition to the use of immunomodulating and biologic agents such as cyclophosphamide and IL-1 receptor antagonists.

Response to steroid treatment is a useful diagnostic tool but only 70% of patients respond to treatment. Delay in treatment beyond 3 months is associated with poor outcomes and potentially irreversible hearing loss.

 Brant JA, Eliades SJ, Ruckenstein MJ. Systematic review of treatments for autoimmune inner ear disease. *Otol Neurotol.* 2015;36(10):1585–92.

Goodall AF, Siddiq MA. Current understanding of the pathogenesis of autoimmune inner ear disease: A review. *Clin Otolaryngol.* 2015;40(5):412–9.

Sudden Sensorineural Hearing Loss

NICHOLAS DAWE

The viva topic will often start by presenting an audiogram in isolation that shows either a unilateral dead ear or an asymmetry. The key is to approach the audiogram in a structured fashion. Consider the presenting symptoms, their timeframe, and if a prior audiogram is available if there is asymmetry. It would be prudent to determine if an asymmetrical loss is new or established.

How would you define sudden sensorineural hearing loss?

'30-3-3': 30 dB sensorineural loss in **three** contiguous frequencies, occurring in under 3 days

This is based on a pure tone audiogram, ideally compared to a previous audiogram. If this is not available, asymmetry must be inferred from the patient's reported symptoms. This is not universally accepted, and various other classifications exist. However, it is useful to be aware of this classification as it is frequently used in research studies.

What are your differential causes?

- Idiopathic: No identifiable cause despite adequate investigation (the majority)
  - Primary autoimmune: Includes autoimmune inner ear disease, may present with bilateral SSNHL, responds to steroids though these may need to be over a prolonged period and require a tapered dose
  - Vascular: AICA stroke (end artery), but likely to be associated with vertigo and cerebellar signs unless only affecting the labyrinthine artery
  - CNS: Multiple sclerosis
  - Viral: Associated with several viral causes, evidence from small studies
  - Infection: Acute labyrinthitis, meningitis, CSOM
  - Intracochlear membrane rupture: May be seen as a first presentation of Ménière's disease
  - Retrocochlear pathology: Vestibular schwannoma
  - Enlarged vestibular aqueduct syndrome, or other cochlear or labyrinthine abnormalities
- Secondary autoimmune conditions
- Systemic causes (including sarcoidosis, hypercoagulability disorders, syphilis, thyroid and cardiovascular disease, diabetes)
- Ototoxic medications: Cisplatin, aminoglycosides and loop diuretics

How would you structure your history?

- Isolated hearing loss?
- Onset and duration, fluctuations. Has there been recurrent hearing loss or any associated neurological impairment?
- Vertigo (30%–40% and poor prognostic factor), dizziness, imbalance, tinnitus
- Ear history: Previous surgery/infections, better hearing ear?
- Trauma, straining, flying, diving – any pressure challenges?
- SH: Key to an ear history are the patient's work and hobbies (noise exposure past, present, future, consequences and safety of hearing loss)
- Cardiovascular status, renal and thyroid disease, diabetes, hypercholesterolaemia
- Autoimmune conditions (GPA, RA, SLE, Cogan syndrome)
- Medication history

How would you approach the case?

Establish the history, perform a complete neurotological examination, including ensuring any middle ear disease is excluded, and performing both a fistula test and tuning fork tests. Consider targeted investigations (bloods if indicated) and undertake an MRI IAMs.

What investigations are indicated and in whom?

A **pure tone audiogram** will have already performed to establish diagnosis. Up sloping and mid-frequency (better) versus down sloping and flat traces (worse).

Bloods: Performing screening blood tests are not recommended by US practice guidelines. If there are specific features in the history, atypical features or if there is a fluctuating or bilateral loss, there may be good reason to perform targeted blood tests.

- Examples include FBC, ESR, autoimmune screen, TFTs, clotting, glucose, VDRL, Lyme serology and HIV.

MRI IAMs: To exclude retrocochlear pathology e.g. vestibular schwannoma

What aspects are important to consider when managing a presumed diagnosis of idiopathic SSNHL?

The cause is unknown at presentation in 85%–90%. Even after thorough investigation, only in one-third it is possible to establish a likely cause. When managing a presumed idiopathic SSNHL, you are likely to be managing a heterogenous group of pathologies, and you should still emphasise that you would approach these cases in a similar fashion. Firstly, a good proportion will resolve without any intervention (32%–65%). Partial hearing improvement or tinnitus would need further assessment, monitoring and support.

Clinical practice guidelines from the United States and the UK are available to support decision making – these are useful to review the summaries. However, there is little robust evidence to support any of the current practice, and to suggest one treatment over another.

National Institute for Health and Care Excellence. Hearing loss in adults: Assessment and management. NICE guideline, 2018. Available at https://www.nice.org.uk/guidance/ng98

How would you manage this patient?

This is best approached in terms of either **primary** or **salvage** treatment.

Consider how you would manage an idiopathic SSNHL if it did not meet criteria, or if referred and an audiogram is not yet available (such as over a weekend). This challenges your knowledge of the evidence and your understanding of the importance of counselling the patient over the risks and benefits of oral steroids.

What are good prognostic factors?

- Time: rapid onset
- Age: younger
- Upsloping audiogram

Is there any evidence for oral steroids over placebo?

There is conflicting evidence for the benefit of steroids, and the latest Cochrane review acknowledged that data is of poor quality and often contradictory. However, it is accepted practice to give early, within 2 weeks and ideally within 72 hours of onset. Limited efficacy is seen after 4–6 weeks. The focus should be on the risk and benefit and patient consent to receiving treatment in the first couple of weeks. Evidence is for low to medium dose (1 mg/kg up to 60 mg maximum for 5–7 days).

What is the evidence for intratympanic (IT) versus oral steroids?

There may be a role for IT therapy, and it may be used regardless of the onset of the hearing loss (up to 3 months). Data shows there is a higher probability of hearing improvement when IT steroids are added as salvage treatment. It may have a role in primary treatment in those who cannot tolerate, or in whom it would not be sensible, to receive oral steroids (diabetic, peptic ulcer, pregnancy, elderly). Therefore, be able to deliver a succinct summary of the risks of a short course of oral steroid therapy. Adverse effects are rare but remain a consideration (e.g. avascular necrosis of the hip).

Do you know of any IT steroids used?

Dexamethasone, methylprednisilone sodium succinate (some evidence of more discomfort when delivered IT)

Other options: Hyperbaric oxygen therapy: No clear evidence for benefit.

How would you follow up a patient with idiopathic SSNHL?

- Investigation by MRI IAMs
- Serial audiograms: Monitor changes and the better hearing ear, assess for progression
- Recommend hearing protection
- Tinnitus therapy

What are your options for hearing rehabilitation?

This is an opportunity to define the issues with single-sided deafness and its impact on hearing in noise and sound localisation. Be able to discuss the benefits of unilateral aid, and in single-sided deafness the role of a CROS/BiCROS aid or a bone conduction hearing implant. CIs are offered for single-sided deafness elsewhere in Europe and worldwide, but within an NHS practice you would have to acknowledge that this is not an option. A CROS aid is considered the most cost-effective option for an individual with a single-sided deafness.

Temporal Bone Fracture

KIRAN JUMANI AND PETER KULLAR

Please describe this image

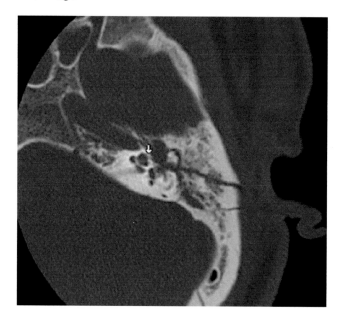

'*This is an axial CT scan of the left temporal bone showing a comminuted fracture which involves the temporal bone passing through the roof of the middle ear*'.

Alternative images may include an otoscopic view of haemotympanum, or Battle's sign (ecchymosis around the mastoid process as a result of extravasation of blood along the path of the posterior auricular artery). This sign usually takes a few days to appear and suggests the patient has sustained a significant injury.

How might they present and how would you manage this patient?

The viva scenario often centres on hearing loss and a sense of aural fullness in a patient with a head injury. Once you are told the patient does not have other neurological symptoms and the neurosurgeons are satisfied there is no other intracranial injury, go through the history and examination systematically. The investigation of choice is high-resolution CT scan of the temporal bone without contrast.

Important elements in history for base of skull fracture:

- Neurological status: Intracranial haematoma/contusion/oedema/herniation (including GCS [Glasgow Coma Scale] assessment)
- Otic capsule/ossicular chain/TM/EAC: Hearing loss and vertigo
- Facial nerve: Immediate or delayed/complete or partial paralysis – valuable prognostic data
- CSF leak: Fistula
- Temporo-mandibular joint injury: Pain/dysfunction
- Lower CN palsies: V-XII
- Jugular vein/carotid artery injury: Potentially catastrophic bleeding

Fractures tend to take the path of least resistance in the bone and follow native foramina. Fractures considered 'open' present with blood, otorrhoea, brain herniation or CSF fistula. These patients are at a higher risk for meningitis as the intracranial space is no longer separated from the environment.

Classification of Temporal Bone Fractures:

Traditionally temporal bone fractures are classified with respect to their orientation to the plane of the petrous ridge. However, this does not provide useful prognostic information with regards to neurotologic deficits.

- **Longitudinal**
- **Transverse**
- **Mixed** (the majority)

A more helpful classification is:

- *Otic capsule sparing*: Caused by a blow to the temporoparietal region. Fracture involves the squamous temporal bone and posterosuperior EAC, running forward through the tegmen tympani and into the region of the facial hiatus. Tend to cause mixed hearing loss or conductive hearing loss.
- *Otic capsule disrupting*: Caused by a blow to the occipital or frontal region. The fracture can run from the foramen magnum across the petrous ridge to the otic capsule, resulting in sensorineural hearing loss and a higher incidence of facial nerve palsy, CSF leak and intracranial complications.

Management:

The initial management of patients with a temporal bone fracture includes the identification and treatment of any life-threatening injuries in conjunction with emergency physicians as appropriate.

Temporal bone fractures usually result from a high-energy impact; therefore, the possibility of an associated intracranial haemorrhage or cervical spine injury is high.

Facial nerve injury:

Facial nerve palsy occurs in 7% of temporal bone fractures. The geniculate ganglion is the commonest site of injury. Decompression of the facial nerve is an area of contention. The key factor in the decision to surgically explore a facial nerve is whether the nerve has a recoverable injury (neuropraxia) or an unrecoverable injury (severed, crushed or impaled with bone fragments).

Patients with delayed onset, complete facial paralysis should be given a 2-week course of systemic corticosteroids (unless medically contraindicated) and observed.

Patients with acute onset, complete facial nerve paralysis should be reassessed around 10 days after the injury to allow for Wallerian degeneration to take place. The degree of injury can be assessed clinically with facial motion and electrodiagnostic tests using the facial nerve stimulator, ENoG or EMG. EMG is the gold standard.

 You may be asked about the interpretation of these electrodiagnostic tests. Patients with a 90% degeneration on ENoG at 14 days may be considered for surgery.

There is a lack of evidence that surgical intervention for an incomplete palsy improves results compared with conservative management, as these patients tend to recover spontaneously. The majority of skull base teams only explore an ear where there is an obvious disruption of the path of the facial nerve or impingement with a bone spicule. The timing of surgical intervention is a point of debate. See the chapter on facial palsy for a further detailed discussion.

Surgery to decompress the facial nerve must expose both the perigeniculate region and the mastoid segment. The transmastoid/supralabyrinthine approach is often used. This approach avoids intracranial exposure and avoids sacrifice of sensorineural hearing; however, it generally requires dislocation of the incus and ossicular reconstruction. Therefore, this approach is ideal in otic capsule sparing fractures with ossicular discontinuity and a well-aerated mastoid. If the patient has any contralateral hearing loss, or the anatomy is not conducive to supralabyrinthine exposure, a middle cranial fossa approach is preferred. The translabyrinthine approach is most often used in otic capsule disrupting fractures.

CSF fistulae: A CSF leak may present as clear otorrhoea if the TM is disrupted or as CSF rhinorrhoea if the TM is intact. Fluid should be sent for Beta 2 transferrin/Beta trace.

Prophylactic antibiotics in the setting of CSF leak is controversial and you may be asked to discuss this in the exam. Meta-analysis does not support the use of prophylactic antibiotics. In otic capsule disrupting fractures, CSF will flow from the posterior fossa into the middle ear through the otic capsule. These fractures are unique in that they do not heal completely. A thin fibrous scar without subsequent enchondral bone formation develops and the patient remains susceptible to meningitis for an indefinite period of time following the injury. Prophylactic pneumococcus, meningococcus and haemophilus vaccination is recommended.

 Ratilal BO, Costa J, Pappamikail L, Sampaio C. Antibiotic prophylaxis for preventing meningitis in patients with basilar skull fractures. *Cochrane Database Syst Rev.* 2015 Apr 28;(4):CD004884. doi: 10.1002/14651858.CD004884.pub4.

Management is generally conservative as the majority of leaks cease spontaneously within 10 days. Surgery may be indicated for persistent leaks (transmastoid or middle fossa approach). See the section on CSF rhinorrhoea in the Rhinology chapter for further details.

Hearing loss: Temporal bone fractures can be associated with conductive hearing loss or mixed sensorineural hearing loss. Otic capsule disrupting fractures cause severe to profound sensorineural hearing loss that is often immediately apparent. Otic capsule sparing fractures can manifest as both sensorineural hearing loss or conductive hearing loss. Conductive hearing loss are caused initially by haemotympanum or effusion, and permanent deficits are caused by disruption of ossicular chain. The most common ossicular chain injuries include subluxation of the incudostapedial joint, dislocation of incus and fracture of stapes crura. Middle ear exploration and ossicular chain reconstruction are considered when a conductive hearing loss persists for more than 2 months post injury. Alternatives to tympanoplasty and ossiculoplasty surgery include air conduction aids, bone conduction devices or CROS aids (in single-sided deafness).

The mechanisms of sensorineural hearing loss are disruption of membranous labyrinth, avulsion or trauma of cochlear nerve, interruption of cochlear blood supply, haemorrhage into the cochlea, perilymph fistula and endolymphatic hydrops resulting from obstruction to endolymphatic duct by the temporal bone fracture. In cases of bilateral dead ear, cochlear implantation should be considered.

Cholesteatoma and external ear canal stenosis:

The pathogenic mechanisms responsible for post-traumatic cholesteatoma formation are:

1. Epithelial entrapment in the fracture line (epitympanum/antrum)
2. In-growth of epithelium through the unhealed fracture line or tear in TM (epitympanum/antrum)
3. Traumatic implantation of TM skin into the middle ear (mesotympanum)
4. Trapping of epithelium medial to a stenosis of the external ear canal (canal cholesteatoma)

Vascular injuries: Intra-temporal carotid artery injury is a rare but life-threatening complication. It is uncommon because the fracture line rarely involves the thick, dense bone surrounding the carotid canal and instead traverses the softer fibrocartilage of the foramen lacerum. The patient may present with bloody otorrhoea and/or neurological signs. In these cases, the ear canal is packed and the patient will need an urgent angiogram and repair with covered stent, balloon occlusion or in extremis, a carotid artery ligation. If there is no active bleeding, CT angiography or MRA can be used to assess the injury.

Tinnitus

NISHCHAY MEHTA

A patient describes hearing an annoying sound in their ear. Describe how you would manage this patient?

'*I would take a directed history focusing on the nature of their symptoms, associated symptoms, risk factors, treatments tried, impact on life, and relevant past medical, drug, social and family history.*

Particularly for a patient presenting with tinnitus I would focus on laterality, onset (e.g. following loud noise exposure), character (pulsatile/clicking/humming/ringing/autophony), alleviating (e.g. digital pressure in neck) and aggravating factors (e.g. quiet, sleep). I would ask about hearing loss, vertigo (especially to loud sounds), otalgia and otorrhoea and previous noise trauma, aspirin or aminoglycoside use. I would ask if it is waking the patient from sleep and how it's impacting on their life.

I would undertake a neurotological examination, auscultate the ear and the neck for bruits, a pure tone audiogram and tympanometry. I would consider ancillary tests depending on the history'.

> The tinnitus viva can take two forms, focussing on either subjective or objective tinnitus. Subjective accounts for 90% of reported cases and describes the perception of a sound in the absence of acoustic, electrical or external stimuli. It is the staple of Otology and General ENT clinics. There is emerging evidence that subjective tinnitus is a result of neuroplastic alterations in the central auditory pathway.

Ninety percent of those with subjective tinnitus have a measurable hearing loss, 50% report laterality to their tinnitus and 10% have intrusive tinnitus. History should focus on the impact of tinnitus on the patient's life. Treatment should be prioritised for patients whose tinnitus has severely impacted their daily lives as they are least likely to improve spontaneously.

Investigations should be aimed at quantifying and classifying any hearing loss. This will help identify patients who warrant further investigations to rule out the more insidious causes of tinnitus (e.g. vestibular schwanommas, Ménière's disease, etc.) and also help direct treatment.

> A viva about subjective tinnitus could focus on a patient who is insistent on a scan so it is useful to have audiometric criteria that would allow you to safely assure a patient that a scan is not necessary. Asymmetry can be classified as 30 dB difference between ears in air conduction thresholds at one frequency, 20 dB difference in averaged thresholds across two consecutive frequencies and 10 dB difference in averaged thresholds across three consecutive frequencies. Patients with symmetrical down sloping mild-moderate sensorineural hearing loss can be assured that further investigations are not <u>currently</u> necessary, but if there is a change in their symptoms of clinical findings then they may become so in the future. The focus of the viva should then be changed to management.

Whilst there is no cure for tinnitus, there are treatments available. Treatments are based on auditory rehabilitation (hearing aids, sound maskers), counselling (CBT, mindfulness) or a combination (tinnitus retraining therapy). Hearing aids are traditionally considered first-line treatment in all patients with a measurable hearing loss. There is considerable variation in treatments offered based on local availability and clinician preference given no gold standard treatment exists.

Objective tinnitus is rare but offers the examiner a chance to explore your understanding of a more surgically relevant aspect of tinnitus.

Causes include:

- Middle ear structures such as myoclonus of tensor tympani and stapedius
- Presence of vascular middle ear tumours (glomus tympanicum)
- Abnormalities of blood vessels that run close to the middle ear or the bone that covers them (Such as arterio-venous malformations and sigmoid sinus dehiscences)
- Eustachian tube and palatal abnormalities (patulous eustachian tube or palatal myoclonus).

How would you manage a patient with superior semicircular canal dehiscence?

'I would confirm their diagnosis through a carefully elicited history, examination, high resolution CT temporal bones and cervical VEMPs. I would counsel them on the potential management options which include conservative strategies of avoiding situations that provoke vertigo symptoms and masking to help with the pulsatile tinnitus and autophony. I would also discuss surgical strategies of resurfacing and plugging of the dehiscence. If they would like to consider surgical treatment, I would refer them to a skull base service where both a mid-cranial fossa and transmastoid approaches can be offered'.

SSCD is frequently accompanied by other vestibular conditions, such as migraines. Optimisation of other vestibular disorders is key to providing the patient with accurate predictions of post-operative outcomes.

Vertigo

NICHOLAS DAWE

The central theme of a vertigo viva will be the extraction of the patient's symptoms in manner facilitating diagnosis. This will necessitate a clear approach to define whether the balance dysfunction occurs due to asymmetry in the labyrinth, vestibular nerve, cerebellum or the central integrators of balance inputs.

Can you classify vertigo symptoms?

There are established definitions; it is important to be able to succinctly summarise a history and formulate a differential.

- Internal: Illusion of own movement of the body, including rotating swaying or tilting
- External: Oscillopsia, illusionary visual movement of the surroundings
- Dizziness: Disturbed perception of spatial orientation without illusionary movement
- Standing and gait instability

What features of the vertigo are you keen to establish from the history?

- Severity, subjective characteristics, intensity and frequency, provoking factors including if positional
- What form does the vertigo take? Horizontal or vertical motion, improvement with eyes opened or closed?
- Accompanying symptoms: Light sensitivity, aural fullness, Tullio phenomenon, syncope, limb weakness
- Supporting information: As for any otological history (associated hearing loss, tinnitus, otalgia, discharge, autophony), previous ear surgery, infections, family history
- Medical comorbidities: Migraine, cardiovascular disease, diabetes, peripheral neuropathy, visual impairment, osteoarthritis including cervical spine restriction, medications
- Impact on daily activities and work

A vertigo viva will be focussed on your understanding of the history and likely common vertigo syndromes, as well as an appreciation of symptoms of the more common peripheral vertigo against a relatively rare central vertigo. This would come in the form of a case presenting to the emergency department and your focus would be on the history and targeted examination. Within this history you would be looking for symptoms of 'vertigo+'. The importance would be to establish a diagnosis that is inconsistent with a peripheral cause and would thus warrant acute medical input.

How would you summarise the integration of balance inputs?

- Visual
- Somatosensory
- Peripheral vestibular
- Sensory integration and the musculoskeletal system

The vestibular system ensures posture and balance adjust in response to gaze and that gaze is stabilised during head tilt (VOR) and rotation (vestibulospinal reflex). Be aware of the range of clinical tests that target these reflexes.

How would you approach the examination?

If the history is not instructive, the neurotological exam becomes essential. A pure tone audiogram and tympanometry are valuable to exclude an asymmetrical hearing loss or middle ear disease. Eye movements and an assessment of the VOR using the head-thrust test can prove highly localising.

Ear examination (including the fistula test), CN assessment including eye movements, tests of cerebellar function, Romberg and Unterberger/Fukuda, gait assessment, and the routine use of Dix–Hallpike test with any history of positional vertigo.

How would you assess eye movements and describe the pattern of nystagmus?

Spontaneous and gaze-evoked nystagmus: Assess in horizontal and vertical planes. Physiological when assessed beyond 30°, so do not assess beyond this degree. The corrective fast phase is away from the affected ear in an acute vestibular loss. Less commonly during an irritative lesion, the fast phase is seen towards the affected ear. It is important to comment that there will be no spontaneous nystagmus in positionally triggered dizziness presentations. Drugs and rare central causes of nystagmus exist including Arnold–Chiari malformations. Failure to suppress with fixation suggests a central origin and thus any assessment of peripheral nystagmus is aided by the use of Frenzel goggles.

 Read about Alexander's law – the amplitude of the nystagmus increases when the eye moves in the direction of the fast phase.

Grade 1 – Nystagmus only in direction of the fast component

Grade 2 – Nystagmus in primary gaze position

Grade 3 – Nystagmus in all eye positions

Smooth pursuit and tests of vergence: Performed by tracking a finger in an arc. Observe for saccades. Whilst problems of smooth pursuit or saccadic eye movements are central in origin, consider age-related change, medication effects, visual acuity and vigilance to the test as factors. Internuclear ophthalmoplegia is pathognomonic of multiple sclerosis.

Halmagyi head-thrust test: Rapid movement of head from midline to 15°–30° to either side whilst asking the patient to fix eyes straight ahead. Observe for overt saccades (inability to keep eyes looking straight ahead) that will occur when tested in the direction of the affected ear. This forms the basis of the vHIT, which can assess for covert corrective saccadic eye movements, in the planes of all six canals.

Head shake: A test of post head-shake nystagmus assessing asymmetry of vestibular tone. The sensitivity of this test is variable. It is performed with rapid oscillation of the head, with or without Frenzel glasses, with eyes closed and asking the patients to open their eyes after 20 seconds. At that moment, whilst continuing to shake the head, observe for nystagmus that will beat towards the stronger side.

Dynamic visual acuity test (DVAT): An objective and behavioural measure of the VOR. Visual acuity is assessed with the head static, then with the head oscillating at 2 Hz either vertically or horizontally – a loss of >3 lines of visual acuity suggests a significant vestibular loss, though is most useful for a bilateral loss.

Hyperventilation test: Hyperventilate for 1 minute – positive if brings on patient's symptoms.

VOR suppression test: The brain is able to suppress the VOR when tracking a moving target with head and eyes moving together. Testing for this involves the patient's arms outstretched and being asked to fixate on thumbs whilst the patient's chair is oscillated. This can also be performed with VNG using a laser light. This is an assessment of the vestibulocerebellum, in particular the flocculus and paraflocculus, although it is a non-specific assessment.

VOG, also known as VNG, is used to record eye movements and assess ocular motor function and the horizontal VOR. The historical form was ENG that used an electrode rather than a video recorder. Be aware of its use in vestibular assessment, as it can be used to formally assess a range of random saccades, smooth pursuit in the horizontal and vertical planes, spontaneous and gaze nystagmus (±fixation), post head-shake nystagmus, positional and positioning tests, bi-thermal calorics, fixation suppression.

Rotational chair testing can provide assessment of the VOR and gives an idea of the patient's compensation. It provides information in the range of 0.01–1 Hz, closer to the frequency of normal head movements (0.01–5 Hz), in contrast to caloric testing that is considered to test lower frequency VOR (0.002–0.004 Hz).

What do Romberg's and Unterberger's/Fukuda's test assess?

Romberg's test: When performed with foam, removes proprioceptive input to reveal any vestibular deficit

Unterberger's/Fukuda's test: Crude and subjective but are intended to assess lateral canal function.

 See Section Examining the 'Dizzy' Patient in Chapter 4.

What can be assessed using caloric testing?

This allows the lateral semicircular canals of both ears to be assessed individually. Caloric irrigation may be performed by water (closed or open loop), or by air irrigation. Typically, bi-thermal caloric irrigation is performed using warm (44°C) or cold (30°C) water. 'COWS' is a reminder that cold elicits an inhibitory and warm an excitatory stimulus (cold water = fast phase of nystagmus to the opposite side as the water filled ear, warm water – fast phase to the same side as the water filled ear). Symmetry of the response and directional preponderance (either a peripheral or central cause) is calculated, with the Jongkee formula employed to determine if a unilateral weakness is present.

If a patient cannot fixate and suppress nystagmus during caloric stimulation, this implies a cerebellar problem.

How else can the VOR be tested?

The VOR may be assessed using frequency-specific tests that assess low- or high-velocity corrections (0.01–1 Hz) (low – caloric, smooth pursuit; high – head thrust, vHIT)

vHIT: This provides side specific information on three-dimensional VOR. The canals are tested in multiple planes of paired canals: horizontal, LARP (left anterior right posterior), RALP (right anterior left posterior), and so this is useful as can be used to assess superior and posterior canal function.

Other tests of balance function

Vestibulospinal reflex: *Posturography* (also referred to as computerised dynamic platform posturography testing) is used to assess the vestibulospinal reflexes, including integration of visual and somatosensory cues. This reflex includes input from the superior SSC and otolithic organs. Various tests are undertaken. They can inform vestibular rehabilitation.

Sensory organisation test: This integrates all aspects. Six conditions and three trials, and an equilibrium score is calculated (0 – fall or step, 100 – no sway). It is an assessment of performance when using somatosensory, visual or vestibular inputs, as well as their ability to ignore conflicting visual inputs.

Otolithic function: *cVEMP*: Unilateral, inhibitory response to an air-click or tone burst stimulus. Requires patient to contract their ipsilateral sternocleidomastoid muscle.

oVEMP (utriculo-ocular, superior vestibular nerve): Excitatory response in contralateral inferior oblique. Less reliable in older patients.

Both useful in the evaluation of suspected superior canal dehiscence syndrome when considering threshold, amplitude and latency of the responses.

What is the role of balance rehabilitation?

Up to 80% see an improvement, with resulting benefit on psychology and quality of life.
Its principles are based on habituation, adaptation, substitution and/or sensory reweighting.

Cawthorne-Cooksey exercises are useful, even in the absence of a cause, for rehabilitating a chronic or poorly compensated imbalance.

Key conditions and their features, and some less common diagnoses, to consider in cases of vertigo

The duration of the vertigo symptoms, precipitating factors and associated otological symptoms should guide you towards a differential. Peripheral vertigo syndromes can often be considered based on duration of symptoms, lasting seconds to minutes, or hours to days, taking into account the more common three pathologies of BPPV, Ménière's disease, and vestibular neuronitis.

Three specific syndromes of vertigo are currently proposed by the Bárány Society, and allow a systematic approach to the symptomatology; these are: (1) acute single episodes of vertigo, (2) episodic conditions that are recurrent in their nature, and, (3) chronic that produce prolonged and persistent vestibular symptoms.

Bisdorff, A.R., Staab, J.P., Newman-Toker, D.E. Overview of the international classification of vestibular disorders. *Neurol Clin.* 2015;33(3):541–550.

Peripheral:

1. Acute vestibular syndromes

- Vestibular neuronitis: Vertigo and gait instability, without the loss of ability to ambulate
- Herpes zoster oticus (Ramsay-Hunt syndrome type 1): A latent herpes zoster affecting the geniculate ganglion. Rare, and associated with a facial palsy (HZV is implicated in 12% of facial palsies, that occur with, or without, a delayed onset of vesicles in the conchal bowl and/or hard palate; evidence exists for corticosteroids alongside antivirals
- Traumatic: Labyrinthine concussion or capsular fractures (risk of labyrinthitis ossificans); if a longitudinal temporal bone fracture occurs with a conductive hearing loss, consider a traumatic perilymphatic fistula (arising from a subluxation of the stapes footplate)

2. Episodic vestibular syndromes

- BPPV: The most frequently encountered cause of vertigo clinically, most commonly affecting the posterior canal (see the section on BPPV)
- Ménière syndrome: Idiopathic (Ménière's disease), post-traumatic, post-infectious (measles, mumps), late stage syphilis (episodic vertigo with a progressive hearing loss), Cogan syndrome
- Benign vertigo of childhood

3. Chronic vestibular syndromes

- Vestibular schwannoma
- Otitis media
- Cholesteatoma and other erosive pathology causing semicircular canal fistulae
- Aminoglycoside toxicity
- Superior canal dehiscence syndrome: Characteristic symptoms of autophony with a variable combination of audiological and vestibular third-window symptoms
- Perilymphatic fistula: Traumatic (fluctuating, progressive, sensorineural or mixed hearing loss, with vertigo precipitated by straining), or 'spontaneous' (a contentious [non-] diagnosis). Difficult to diagnose; Cochlin-Tomoprotein is a recently proposed biomarker.

Central:

1. Acute vestibular syndromes

- Brainstem ischaemia
- Transient ischaemic attack: Rotational vertebral artery syndrome (neutral and symptomatic vascular imaging)

- PICA stroke: Wallenberg syndrome (lateral medullary syndrome), can be traumatic when precipitated by preceding trauma or neck pain
- AICA stroke: Second most common brainstem stroke, with variable effect on hearing, including labyrinthine infarction (perhaps more of a peripheral cause as only causes hearing loss), internal auditory artery occlusion, a branch of the AICA causing an abrupt vertigo and tinnitus; proximal AICA stroke affecting lateral pons and cerebellar peduncle – facial paralysis, gait and limb ataxia and vertigo with hearing loss
- Cerebellar infarction and haemorrhage: Similar to peripheral acute neuritis but nystagmus towards, and unable to stand, falling towards the lesion; impaired smooth pursuit

2. Episodic vestibular syndromes

- Vestibular migraine: Recurrent vestibular symptoms, without hearing loss, and a migraine aura that can frequently occur without a headache. Response to standard migraine therapies supports the diagnosis.
- Episodic ataxia type 2

 Be aware of the definitions of migrainous vertigo and the criteria to diagnose, proposed by Neuhauser.

3. Chronic vestibular syndromes

- MS: Peripheral or central form depending on the location of the plaques
- Arnold–Chiari malformation: Positional nystagmus that resolves with head movement (down-beating nystagmus)
- Mal de debarquement (MdDS): Rocking, bobbing, or swaying, following passive motion stimulus, that occurs up to 1 month following the exposure. MdDS is worse when a patient is not moving, and improvements often occur when returning to motion, typically driving (>80%). There is often a history of recent cruise, or similar low-frequency motion exposure, of 1 week or more. Vestibular rehabilitation, in the form of VOR modulation, is considered to aid remission.
- Persistent Postural-Perceptual Dizziness: A chronic functional disorder of non-vertiginous dizziness lasting 3 months or more. Distinct from psychiatric causes of vestibular disorders and is a maladaptation disorder of balance control and vestibular processing precipitated by an acute or chronic vestibular or balance-related problem (in contrast to MdDS). Symptoms are worse when upright and exacerbated by visual stimuli and either active or passive head movements. Now recognised as a maladaptive state, patients were previously likely grouped into phobic postural vertigo, space motion discomfort, visual vertigo, or chronic subjective dizziness. Patient information, vestibular rehabilitation, physiotherapy, medication and CBT, all thus offer therapeutic opportunities to escape from the maladaptive cycle.

Other considerations

- Consider how to respond to 'dizziness' presenting in childhood. BPPV is not reported in children under 11 years of age and the importance of the history, including parental and patient anxieties, should be emphasised, before embarking on extensive balance assessment and targeted imaging.

Understand the role of MRI in an acute stroke: Diffusion (non-contrast) useful at 30 minutes – 5 days; FLAIR sequences (1 day – months); T1 contrast enhanced (5 days – 2 months). The immediate clinical assessment is invaluable.

- The HINTS acronym: head impulse, nystagmus type, test of skew is a highly effective three-component eye battery clinical test that is more sensitive than MRI in the first 2 days of a stroke.

Blood tests may be indicated in cases of suspected systemic causes.

How would you differentiate a central from a peripheral cause?

It is useful to have in mind what features differentiate a central from a peripheral cause, when given a history of an acute vertigo. Patients with Ménière's disease do not typically present to an emergency department. The challenge is to identify any concerning features that represent an impending medical emergency or identify BPPV or a more benign cause.

Features of a peripheral origin include a spontaneous nystagmus with a fixed direction that is both horizontal and suppressed by fixation, the absence of skew deviation (be able to outline this), a positive HIT, reduced DVAT, and imbalance without ataxia.

Risk factors for a central cause of acute vertigo might include the inability to stand unassisted, an associated hearing loss, and any 'vertigo plus' presentations representing an acute stroke. Any incoordination with neurological symptoms, spontaneous nystagmus that is enhanced with fixation, abnormal smooth pursuit, saccadic eye movements, positional nystagmus that is atypical, skew deviation, normal HIT and an ataxic gait. An evolving stroke gives the patient lateral propulsion and so they will not be able to stand unassisted.

COMMON PAEDIATRIC ENT VIVA TOPICS

EDITED BY BENJAMIN HARTLEY AND RICHARD J HEWITT

7

- Branchial anomalies
- Cervical lymphadenopathy
- Choanal atresia
- Cleft lip and palate
- Congenital midline nasal masses
- Developmental milestones, hearing and speech, autism
- Drooling
- Juvenile nasopharyngeal angiofibroma
- Laryngomalacia
- Microtia
- Obstructive sleep apnoea
- Otitis media
- Paediatric airway compromise
- Paediatric hearing loss
- Periorbital cellulitis
- Recurrent respiratory papillomatosis
- Syndromes in ENT
- Thyroglossal duct cyst
- Tonsillitis and post-tonsillectomy bleeding
- Vascular malformations

Branchial Anomalies

JESSICA BEWICK

A 4-year-old child presents to your clinic with hearing loss. During your examination you notice a small pit in the right side of the neck. On further questioning the child's mother tells you that this has been present since birth and that it discharges on occasion but seems to cause no distress. Palpation reveals a small sinus along the anterior border of the sternocleidomastoid (junction upper 2/3 and lower 1/3) with no underlying mass.

What is the likely diagnosis?

Second branchial cleft sinus

> While one could arrange an ultrasound to confirm, a discharging sinus in this position is pathognomonic of a second branchial cleft anomaly and unless there is an underlying mass or history of neck swelling, it is not required.

> Second branchial cleft sinuses/cysts/fistulas make up around 90% of branchial anomalies.

What is the embryological origin of this anomaly?

The sinus tract contains skin originating from the ectodermal layer of the second branchial cleft. While the cleft at this level usually obliterates as the operculum descends over the third and fourth clefts during the fifth week of embryological development, it can leave an ectodermal remnant responsible for branchial cysts and fistulae. The extent of the tract can be blind ending or a true fistula connected to the palatine tonsil, passing in between the external and internal carotid arteries on its way.

What treatment would you offer?

'A discharging neck sinus is unpleasant and carries the risk of infection. I would therefore offer surgical excision as a definitive treatment'.

In the appropriately consented, anaesthetised and positioned patient I would:

- Gently explore with a lacrimal probe (ensuring not to make false tract)
- Perform an elliptical incision around the sinus
- Dissect onto the tract with the probe *in situ* (held by an Allis clamp if required)
- Be aware the tract may have cystic dilatations
- Follow the tract up to the bifurcation of the carotid or pharynx if necessary
- Tie the base with a vicryl suture
- Be prepared to make a step-ladder incision if required

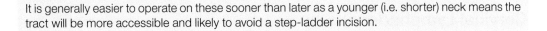

It is generally easier to operate on these sooner than later as a younger (i.e. shorter) neck means the tract will be more accessible and likely to avoid a step-ladder incision.

If connected to the tonsil, should this be removed?

This used to be advised but most surgeons have moved away from this step as it does not seem to provide therapeutic advantage (and may instead introduce added risk of haemorrhage).

Given the initial presentation of hearing loss, if this was not due to OME would you be concerned about any syndromes?

Yes, both hearing loss (conductive, sensorineural or mixed) and second branchial cleft anomalies are major criteria of branchio-oto-renal syndrome. I would examine for other abnormalities (e.g. preauricular pits etc.), enquire about family history (autosomal dominant with variable penetrance) and ensure the child was referred for a renal USS and to a paediatrician/geneticist for further assessment.

Can you tell me about first branchial cleft anomalies and how are they classified?

First branchial cleft cysts are congenital cysts occuring in the parotid, submandibular or preauricular region and a remnant of the first branchial cleft. They have been classified by Work (1972):

- Type 1: Runs from the auricular area parallel to the EAC (ectodermal)
  - Wide excision of the tract including cartilage is the typical surgical option
- Type 2: Typically found at the anterior neck skin above the hyoid (ectodermal and mesodermal)
  - Can run over the mandible and through parotid (beware the facial nerve) towards the bony-cartilaginous EAC junction
  - Varied presentation: pre-auricular sinus, EAC swelling (always examine the ear canal) and discharge, sinus or abscess along the mandible (consider the differential of atypical mycobacterial infection)
  - CT/MRI/sinogram may help identify relationship to the facial nerve
  - Surgery involves a parotidectomy approach

Beware that there is no reliable clinical or radiological method of differentiating types 1 and 2 so surgeons should always be aware that the tract may course deep to the facial nerve.

Third and fourth branchial pouch anomalies:

- Always left-sided, tracking from the neck to the pyriform fossa
- Present with recurrent thyroiditis or an anterior neck abscess
- Barium swallow is helpful in the diagnosis
- Surgical options include tract excision possibly with hemithyroidectomy or direct endoscopy and application of diathermy/tissue glue to the pyriform fossa opening

Cervical Lymphadenopathy

JESSICA BEWICK

A mother brings her 11-year-old daughter to see you with a lump in the right side of her neck. What would you do in clinic?

Cervical lymphadenopathy is a common presentation to the ENT clinic and candidates are expected to have an evidence-based approach to appropriately investigate children. Your role is primarily to identify those children who have disease other than reactive lymphadenopathy which affects almost all children at some stage.

History important points

- Lump duration, size, fluctuation and skin changes (the most significant symptom is progressive enlargement)
- Systemic features e.g. B-type symptoms
- History of recurrent tonsillitis and URTIs
- Previous history of malignancy
- Foreign travel, pets and TB contacts

Examination important points

- Lump size, region, overlying skin
- Other lumps
- Tonsils – for current infection +/– asymmetry
- Ears and nose for disease (infective source, primary tumour)
- Hepatosplenomegaly

There is a 2.5-cm firm lump in the right level 2 region with healthy overlying skin. This has been slowly enlarging over the last 6 weeks. Smaller lumps can be felt adjacent to this. The child is otherwise well, normal examination with no risk factors for TB. What would your next step be?

'A lump of 2 cm or more in a well child (particularly without history of recurrent URTIs) is concerning for a malignant process involving a lymph node. I would obtain a USS of the neck (to

assess nodal size and architecture) along with serological blood tests for EBV, Toxoplasma, and Bartonella alongside an FBC and CRP. I would also arrange a chest X-ray. Serological testing can be positive in up to 10% of patients and may prevent the need for open biopsy. Due to the size of the lump and in line with current evidence I would organise urgent biopsy of the lymph node. I would also liaise with colleagues in paediatric oncology who may want to meet with the patient prior to biopsy and inform the histopathologist of the date the biopsy is anticipated'.

If questioned on the urgency of the requested biopsy, one could state that it can take a few days to find a theatre slot; in the meantime, the other investigations can be completed which can then be reviewed and if necessary the need for biopsy reconsidered should a non-malignant diagnosis seem more likely.

Why would you do an ultrasound if you are going to take out the node anyway?

The ultrasound would give information about the nodal size and architecture and importantly if it is contained within a confluence of lymph nodes, this may change my surgical approach to a wedge nodal biopsy instead of full excision. Due to the risks of operating within this region with relation to the marginal mandibular nerve in particular, surgical planning is paramount. In addition, while this is most likely to be a lymph node, it is possible a firm lump in the level 2 region is another pathology which again may change surgical management.

Why proceed to open biopsy rather than an FNA-c?

The primary concern in a child of this age is of lymphoma. Diagnosis is based upon histological analysis of preferably a whole node. Whilst FNA-c is useful in adults to exclude SCC, this is not reliable in this age group. A core biopsy is an alternative, although this may not also be available or appropriate for a young child.

Lymphoma is the third commonest malignancy in children and the most common in the head and neck region.

What is the differential diagnosis?

- Reactive hyperplasia secondary to infection including EBV
- Metastatic lymph node
- Branchial cyst (although would expect the lump to be fluctuant)
- Rhabdomyosarcoma
- Neurofibroma

 This is a must-read paper that summarises current UK paediatric ENT practice:

Locke R, Comfort R, Kubba H. 'When does an enlarged cervical lymph node in a child need excision? A systematic review'. *International Journal of Pediatric Otorhinolaryngology* 2014;78(3):393–401.

Choanal Atresia

MATTHEW ELLIS

You are asked to see a neonate who was delivered without complication earlier in the day. She is noted to have noisy breathing, signs of respiratory distress and difficulty feeding. An attempt to pass an NG tube was unsuccessful.

What is the differential diagnosis for nasal obstruction with dyspnoea in neonates?

- Choanal atresia
- Pyriform aperture stenosis
- Encephalocele
- Dermoid cyst
- Benign nasal tumour
- Nasolacrimal duct cyst
- Turbinate hypertrophy

Describe congenital choanal atresia

'Bilateral congenital choanal atresia is a rare (1 in 7,000 live births) life-threatening airway emergency which presents within the first few hours of life with acute respiratory distress and feeding difficulties. Two-thirds of cases are unilateral and may present later in life'.

Important elements in the history

- Short duration of feeding
- Cyclical cyanosis (breathing improves on crying)
- Increased work of breathing, intercostal recession
- Rhinorrhoea

How would you assess nasal patency at the bedside?

- Cold spatula test
- Airflow detection with a stethoscope
- Ability to pass NG tube (size 8F)
- Flexible nasendoscopy

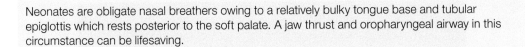

Neonates are obligate nasal breathers owing to a relatively bulky tongue base and tubular epiglottis which rests posterior to the soft palate. A jaw thrust and oropharyngeal airway in this circumstance can be lifesaving.

Which syndromes are associated with choanal atresia?

- CHARGE (coloboma, heart defects, atresia choanae, restricted growth, genital abnormality, ear defects)
- Treacher Collins syndrome
- Apert syndrome
- DiGeorge syndrome
- VACTERL association (vertebral, anorectal, cardiovascular abnormalities, tracheoesophageal fistula, oesophageal atresia, renal abnormalities, limb defects)
- Trisomy 18 (Edwards syndrome)

Several of these syndromes are characterised by midline defects. About 50% of patients with congenital choanal atresia have a recognised syndrome. The most common is CHARGE which is present in 25%.

What is the embryology of this condition?

Different theories exist: persistence of the buccopharyngeal membrane or nasobuccal membrane. Whilst previously divided into membranous and bony types, the vast majority are now known to be mixed.

Which investigations would you undertake?

- Flexible nasendoscopy
- CT scan
- Microlaryngoscopy

CT provides information on whether the defect is bony or membranous, unilateral or bilateral and whether there are additional airway lesions. The nose should be suctioned to clear secretions immediately before the scan.

If indicated, investigation for the underlying cause should be performed in conjunction with the paediatricians e.g. renal USS/ECG/echo. If there are syndromic features clinical genetics should be involved.

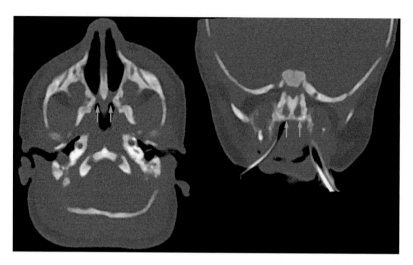

How would you initially manage this condition?

'This is a potential airway emergency. Secretions need to be suctioned from the nose. Supplemental oxygen should be applied and saturations monitored. An oropharyngeal airway should be used to keep the airway open until definitive management is undertaken'.

Describe a surgical technique to treat choanal atresia

- Boyle-Davis gag
- 120° Hopkins endoscope to visualise nasopharynx
- Topical nasal decongestion
- Perforate medial side of atretic plate with urethral dilator
- Increase lumen with drill, serial dilations or balloon (membranous only)

Whilst some surgeons have recommended excising the vomer and medial pterygoid plate to reduce risk of restenosis, others suggest that preserving the vomer in bilateral choanal atresia helps stents remain in the correct position to stabilise the airway and feeding.

Variations on the technique include use of a drill, microdebrider or balloon dilation. Open techniques have been almost entirely replaced by endoscopic techniques.

Would you insert a stent?

There is variation in practice around the country regarding this. Say what you would do.

A 2015 meta-analysis showed that stent insertion did not prevent restenosis rates but was associated with a higher rate of complications such as septal necrosis, synechiae and displacement.

However, some units use stents in order to better stabilise the airway and feeding.

There is insufficient published literature on mitomycin C.

Strychowsky JE, Kawai K, Moritz E et al. To stent or not to stent? A meta-analysis of endonasal congenital bilateral choanal atresia repair. *Laryngoscope.* 2016 Jan;126(1):218–27.

What are the complications of surgery?

- Re-stenosis – the most common complication
- Septal perforation or alar necrosis from stents
- Base of skull injury

Cleft Lip and Palate

SUNIL SHARMA

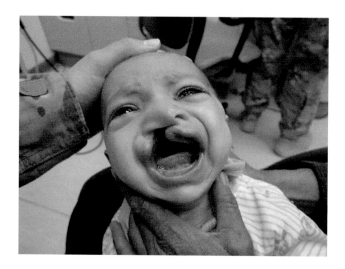

What is the diagnosis in this photograph?

'*This is a clinical photograph of a child with unilateral complete cleft lip and palate (Veau Group III)*'.

Describe the developmental abnormality relevant to this condition

The embryonic face is formed by the fusion of the frontonasal prominence, the paired right and left maxillary prominence and the right and left mandibular prominences.

- Week 4: Pharyngeal arch formation, first pharyngeal arch contributes to the mandible and maxilla
- Weeks 6–7: Primary palate formation, maxillary processes and frontonasal prominence form the lip and alveolus
- Week 9: Secondary palate shelves fuse, separating oral and nasal cavities (palate is fused by week 12)

Disruption of any of these phases of development contributes to cleft lip and palate formation and this can be diagnosed in the second trimester by a USS.

Are you aware of any classification systems associated with this condition?

Cleft palate can be described as primary (anterior) or secondary (posterior) depending on its position relative to the incisive foramen.

Different classification systems exist but a commonly used one for cleft palate is the Veau classification system:

- Incomplete soft palate – Veau Group I
- Incomplete hard palate – Veau Group II
- Unilateral complete lip and palate – Veau Group III
- Bilateral complete lip and palate – Veau Group IV

In addition to these types a submucous cleft palate is where the palate appears grossly intact without a cleft. However, deep to the mucosa there may be separation of the levator palatini muscles and hence a dysfunctional palate. Signs include a midline palate translucent area (zona pellucida), bifid uvula and a notched hard palate. It is important to always to inspect the palate if an adenoidectomy is proposed.

Classification for cleft lip:

- Unilateral complete/incomplete
- Bilateral complete

 Read about the LAHSHAL notation system for cleft lip and palate.

What syndromes are associated with this condition?

Cleft lip and palate can be isolated (50%–60%) or associated with syndromes such as:

- Pierre Robin sequence
- Treacher Collins syndrome
- Velocardiofacial syndrome (6%–8%)
- Goldenhar syndrome
- Van der Woude syndrome

Which members are present in an MDT cleft clinic?

- Cleft surgeon
- ENT surgeon
- Geneticist
- Cleft specialist nurse
- Craniofacial consultant
- Audiologist
- Orthodontist
- Dentist
- Psychologist
- Speech and language therapist

What risk factors are associated with development of this condition?

- Maternal alcohol consumption
- Smoking
- Anticonvulsant use
- Previous cleft child
- Family history of cleft

What are the ENT issues associated with this condition?

- Airway: Options include nasopharyngeal airways, CPAP and tracheostomy depending on the underlying syndrome
- Speech: SLT essential, pharyngoplasty a surgical option
- Feeding to identify: Haberman feeder, NG top-ups; essential to be comfortable with the different types of teats available for cleft patients as you may be asked about them/ identify them (e.g. MAM and NUK teats)
- Hearing: These children need regular hearing assessment. They are at higher risk of OME. The NICE guidance suggests grommets should be offered as an alternative to hearing aids but this doesn't necessarily need to be done at the same time as cleft repair. Be up to speed with the latest guidance (NICE CG60).
- Otological: There is a higher risk of cholesteatoma and chronic otitis media

Describe the timeline for management of this condition

Remember the Rule of 10s.

• Cleft lip – repair at 10 weeks if Hb >10 and weight >10 lbs, need special teat due to feeding problems
- Cleft palate – repair at 10 months (can do grommets at the same time for difficulties in hearing and speech development)
- Columellar lengthening at 5 years
- Orthodontic procedures 8–16 years
- Dental implants and alveolar bone grafting 10 years
- Midface advancement and rhinoplasty 16 years

What are the options if you discover evidence of a submucosal cleft intra-operatively prior to undertaking an adenoidectomy?

- Limited/partial adenoidectomy by suction diathermy leaving a central band of tissue against the soft palate to reduce the risk of velopharyngeal insufficiency in the text
- Abandon the operation and refer to Cleft MDT clinic

Congenital Midline Nasal Masses

SUNIL SHARMA

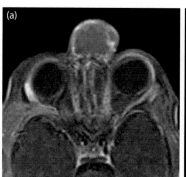 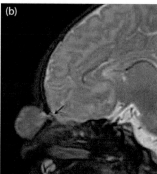

Please describe the scan above

'*This is a T1-weighted axial (a) and T2-weighted sagittal MRI (b) that demonstrates a non-enhancing midline nasal mass that may have a potential intracranial connection with the anterior cranial fossa as denoted by the arrow*'.

This is a common exam scenario with three clear differentials, all of which you should be familiar with.

What is your differential diagnosis?

- Nasal glioma (consists of dysplastic glial cells without an intracranial connection)
- Nasal dermoid (formed by trapped ectodermal elements in the prenasal space during embryonic development)
- Nasal encephalocele (neural tube defect with herniation of cranial contents through the anterior skull base into the nasal area)

What pertinent questions would you ask in the history?

- Increase in size of the mass when patient cries or strains (suggests nasal encephalocele)
- Any history of meningitis

What would you look for on examination?

- A midline lump on dorsum or glabella +/− associated punctum which secretes sebum/fluid suggests a nasal dermoid

- Hair emerging from punctum is pathognomic of nasal dermoid
- Furstenberg sign – compression of IJV causes increase in size of an encephalocele

What further investigations would you perform?
- If rhinorrhoea is present, test for beta-2 transferrin
- CT scan of the sinuses and brain (to assess for any bony defect)

What management options are available?

If nasal dermoid:

- Superficial lesions managed with a nasofrontal incision with eyebrow extensions
- If intraosseous tract, will require either external septorhinoplasty approach or endonasal rhinoplasty approach
- Access to skull base via medial osteotomies and burr drill
- Intracranial extension managed with bicoronal flap and craniotomy, or brow incision and anterior small craniotomy

If nasal encephalocele:

- Need to establish if basal or vault encephaloceles.
- They are further classified as anterior (sincipital) or posterior (occipital).
- Anterior encephaloceles: Transethmoidal, transsphenoidal, transorbital and interfrontal or frontoethmoidal (often present with mass on lateral nose which transilluminates). Posterior encephaloceles range from a skin blemish (cephalocele) to giant encephaloceles.
- Surgical options include endoscopy with repair of skull base defect with fascia lata and fat graft, or craniotomy and repair of dura.

If nasal glioma:

- Establish whether tissue is present extranasally, intranasally or between the nose and the lateral nasal wall through bone (or rarely, with intracranial extension).
- Intranasal gliomas can be removed endoscopically. Extranasal gliomas can be excised through a skin incision.

Developmental Milestones, Hearing and Speech, Autism

JESSICA BEWICK

Assessing developmental milestones can fill the general ENT surgeon with dread, particularly in the child with complex medical needs. However, anyone who is assessing and treating children (in particular those with hearing loss) should have a basic framework of developmental progress in order to identify those who may have other related conditions.

A 3-year-old boy is seeing you in clinic with his mother for concerns about hearing loss. You ask about the usual history which identifies normal newborn hearing screen, hearing concerns since 2 years of age and three to four ear infections per year usually with URTIs. His mother mentions his very limited vocabulary compared to his peers. By 3 years old what basic communication skills would you expect him to have?

 • Three-word sentences
- Knows some colours
- Knows his name + age
- Able to follow at least two-step commands

You test this in clinic – he is only able to name basic objects (juice, car). He will follow a one-step request for his mother. You have difficulty engaging with him, there is no eye contact or attempt to communicate with you or the nurse directly. What are your thoughts?

Naming common objects and one-step requests are usually developed by the age of 18 months so he has a significant developmental delay. While some children are shy in new environments, they will have developed good eye contact in their first year and are usually inquisitive and interactive by this age.

'I would want to ask the mother further questions about social interaction and check other developmental milestones such as age first sat/crawled/walked/babbled/first words (6–8 months/8–9 months/13 months/3 months/10 months respectively). If I identify a social and emotional developmental delay I would want to get a full audiological history'.

His gross motor and initial speech development raised no concerns. He often seems to ignore his immediate family and has the TV volume up loud. Any words he knows are often repeated as are some behaviours. His mother is upset as she has been told by family members that he may have autism but she feels this is primarily a hearing issue. How would you test his hearing?

- If possible, a full ENT examination
- Usually at the age of 3, play audiometry would be appropriate

- Inability to follow two-step instructions prevents this, in which case refer for visual-reinforced audiometry
- Tympanometry

Developmental milestones dictate the type of hearing test that can be employed at each age:

- Startle (up to 6 months)
  - Basic reflexes e.g. changing facial expression/pupil dilatation/crying observation
- VRA (7 months to ~2.5 years)
  - Ability to turn head 180° (4 months for fix and follow)
  - Sit upright (6 [unsupported] – 8 [supported] months)
  - Auditory localisation strongly influenced by visual reinforcement
- Play audiometry (~2 years to ~5 years)
  - Ability to follow two-step commands (hear sound then do play task)
  - Gross motor skills appropriate (usually sit unaided, reaching)
  - Fine motor skills appropriate (from basic placing object in bucket to jigsaw puzzle)

You review the child back in clinic after VRA which shows a very borderline free-field hearing loss and type B tymp on the left, type C on the right. Audiology will repeat this in 3 months. Mum is reassured that all his problems could be due to the eustachian tube dysfunction. The child continues to have limited communication skills, is upset in clinic but refuses affection from mum and has repetitive behaviour. What would you say?

- Need to highlight to the parents that social interaction and communication skills are far below that expected
- There is concern regarding autism spectrum disorder due to features of repetitive behaviour, lack of eye contact etc.
- Referral to a community paediatrician for further assessment is essential

Any healthcare professional caring for children should act in their best interest and in such circumstances it is entirely appropriate to refer on to a specialist for such symptoms. Not doing so (or at the very least highlighting concerns to the GP) could be considered negligent.

What methods of reducing stress for children with ASD who are undergoing surgery do you know?

- Morning surgery
- Starve appropriately for the planned theatre time
- Inform anaesthetist and consider pre-med
- Aim for day case surgery when possible and discharge early when safe
- Introduce a calm quiet environment

Drooling

GARETH LLOYD

This is a classic example of a common condition where you can score very highly with a little preparation. However, you will score poorly if it is clear you have never managed such a child or fail to present the management options in a logical stepwise manner.

It is essential to distinguish a scenario depicting chronic salivary incontinence (discussed here) from an acutely drooling child which may indicate an upper airway emergency.

You are shown an image of a child with moisture, erythema and excoriation over her chin suggestive of chronic excessive drooling. What is drooling and how would you measure its severity?

Drooling is the unintentional loss of saliva from the mouth. It is a normal phenomenon in many children prior to the development of oral neuromuscular control at age 18–24 months but considered abnormal if it persists beyond the age of 4 years. Drooling may be caused by overproduction of saliva (rare, except for when teething) or decreased clearance (common). The most likely aetiology to require active management is the lack of neuromuscular coordination (20%–30% of children with cerebral palsy have problematic drooling). These children have a poor swallowing reflex with reduced oromotor and lingual control. Your history and examination should aim to elucidate the aetiology and severity of the condition with these differentials in mind.

Severity can be established through the number of bib/clothing changes per day and the incidence of peri-oral skin breakdown. The psychological effects on the child and parents' well-being should also be considered and can be captured using validated symptom questionnaires.

Where is saliva produced?

The salivary glands are under parasympathetic control and secrete 1–1.5 L of saliva per day. The submandibular glands is primarily responsible for resting secretions (70%), the parotid responds to food excitation (25%) and the sublingual glands contribute approximately 5%.

Recall that the parasympathetic innervation of the parotid is distinct to that of the submandibular and sublingual glands: The parotid gland is supplied by CNIX; the submandibular and sublingual glands are supplied by CNVII.

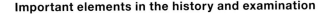

Important elements in the history and examination

Always include an account of the perinatal period and the child's general developmental progress. This should uncover significant neuromuscular issues. It is essential to determine whether the child is at high risk of aspiration as this will impact both the urgency for treatment and the appropriate management option. You also need to know if this condition is stable or likely to improve/deteriorate.

In an otherwise healthy child, briefly explore causes of salivary overproduction such as teething, medications (e.g. nitrazepam used for seizures), GORD, liver disease, pancreatitis, oral ulceration and infection.

A complete head and neck exam is required. Note the head position and movement; viscosity of secretions; lip seal; dentition and occlusion; tongue size and mobility; tonsillar hypertrophy (obstructing swallowing) and adenoidal hypertrophy (mouth breathing). Verbalise to the examiner that the child is wearing a bib or has peri-oral excoriation.

What investigations would you undertake?

In reality you may not request any investigations but involve the wider MDT consisting of SLT, paediatricians (neurology and respiratory) and dental services. All children should undergo evaluation of their oromotor function with SLT. Barium swallow, FEES and nuclear medicine salivagrams may be indicated in certain patients. Ultrasound is typically not necessary.

How would you manage this condition?

'I manage drooling in a stepwise manner depending on the severity, underlying cause and response to prior interventions. Broadly, it can be managed by non-surgical or surgical means but my first line is always SLT for assessment and oro-motor therapy. The vast majority of children with normal neurodevelopment require no additional intervention. Medical management is limited by the side effects of systemic anticholinergic treatment but reflux can be addressed. Botulinum toxin (A) can be injected into the submandibular glands, parotid or both. At my institution, we inject both submandibular glands under ultrasound guidance and typically repeat this at 6 months'.

When would you to proceed to surgery?

Surgical options include relocation of the submandibular ducts, ligation of the ducts, excision of the submandibular glands or tympanic neurectomy. Relocation of the duct posteriorly is contraindicated if there is an unsafe swallow with high risk of aspiration. Ligation of the submandibular ducts does not appear to cause gland swelling in the same way as performing parotid duct ligation. Excising the glands is effective but leaves two scars in the neck and risks injury to the marginal mandibular and lingual nerves. Tympanic neurectomy is limited as it only reduces innervation to the parotid (less important for resting salivation) and is now only of historical interest.

How do you perform relocation of the submandibular duct?

Dissect an island of mucosa in the floor of the mouth and develop this posteriorly towards the lingual nerves. Create a submucosal tunnel each side to the base of the tonsil and pass each duct through. Secure this in place with suture. Complete the operation with excision of the sublingual gland to avoid ranula formation (see the Ranula chapter in the Head and Neck section of this book).

Juvenile Nasopharyngeal Angiofibroma

COLIN BUTLER

In this scenario, you will often be presented a brief clinical history of epistaxis and nasal obstruction in an adolescent male.

What other history is relevant?

Your history should be as for any epistaxis history, with a focus on duration, laterality and failed courses of treatment. JNA will often present with nasal obstruction (80%) but also epistaxis (50%), headache (25%) and facial swelling (15%). Ask about eye symptoms and signs (diplopia, proptosis) and unilateral otological symptoms (OME). Examiners may volunteer examination findings of a unilateral nasal mass.

Opening questions may alternatively start with the initial management of epistaxis and work towards a unilateral mass.

What is the differential diagnosis and how would you investigate this further?

'My differential for this nasal mass would include a benign nasal polyp, an inverted papilloma, a teratoma, an encephalocele, nasal dermoid and rare neoplastic processes such as a nasopharyngeal cancer, an olfactory neuroblastoma or a rhabdomyosarcoma. The history of recurrent epistaxis makes a differential of juvenile nasopharyngeal highly likely. I would further investigate this with cross-sectional imaging of the paranasal sinuses with a CT and an MRI'.

The following images are from investigations performed for the nasal mass. Please describe them

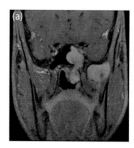 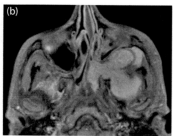 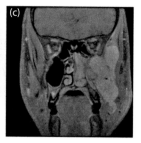

'These are axial (b) and coronal (a and c) T1 fat-saturated post-gadolinium MRI scans of the paranasal sinuses, demonstrating an enhancing tumour in the left nasal cavity nasopharynx and sphenoid. Notably on the axial scan, the tumour can be seen widening the left sphenopalatine foramen and extending into the infratemporal fossa. The coronal scans show evidence of tumour eroding and expanding the left vidian canal and foramen rotundum'.

Characteristic features to mention:

> • CT: Marked contrast enhancement; anterior bowing of the posterior maxillary wall (Holman–Miller sign)
> • Widening of the pterygomaxillary fissure and pterygopalatine fossa; widening of the sphenopalatine foramen as the tumour 'dumbbells' through
> • MRI: Better at defining orbital and intracranial extension. T2 images may show features of flow void loops (salt-and-pepper appearance; salt = punctate hyperintense regions, pepper = small flow voids)

Note that salt-and-pepper appearance is classically seen in paragangliomas (typically on T1) whereas in JNA more seen in T2 images.

This will be an opportunity to highlight a staging system. The examiner may ask this as a separate question.

How would you stage this disease?

Fisch staging system:

- Stage I: Limited to the nasopharyngeal cavity; bone destruction negligible or limited to the sphenopalatine foramen
- Stage II: Invading the pterygopalatine fossa or the maxillary, ethmoid or sphenoid sinus with bone destruction
- Stage III: Invading the infratemporal fossa or orbital region (A) without intracranial involvement or (B) with intracranial extradural (parasellar) involvement
- Stage IV: Intracranial intradural tumour (A) without infiltration of the cavernous sinus, pituitary fossa or optic chiasm, or (B) with infiltration of the cavernous sinus, pituitary fossa or optic chiasm

 Be aware of other staging systems, which include Radkowski/Chandler/Andrews/UPMC (all have a very similar method of classification).

How would you manage this child?

Surgery is the mainstay of management.

Medical management includes hormonal treatment with finasteride (testosterone inhibitor) but this is infrequently used.

RT is reserved for tumours considered unresectable (rare), however side effects in adolescents are considerable. These include retarded growth, temporal lobe necrosis and sarcomatous transformation. RT is therefore discouraged where possible.

What are the surgical approaches?

Surgery can be endoscopic or open. Typically stage I and II disease is managed via an endoscopic approach. Stage III and IV disease is managed via an open approach. Increasingly stage III disease have been attempted endoscopically. A combined approach can also be considered. Regardless of technique, tumour should be fully resected. Open approaches include lateral rhinotomy, transfacial, transpalatal and infratemporal fossa. Midfacial degloving is used in many units as it gives considerable access.

Examiners may ask why you might use one technique over another. Be prepared to discuss other techniques. Highlight the principles of surgery, namely adequate access, lateral to medial dissection and adequate removal to prevent recurrence. Some surgeons advocate drilling the pterygoid (vidian) canal. Surgery is often combined with preoperative embolisation.

What precautions would you take before surgery?

Bleeding is significant during this operation and workup would include the possibility of embolisation.

Be prepared to discuss the pros and cons.

- Pros: Reduces blood loss (2-fold), improves visualisation of operative anatomy.
- Cons: Embolic events (stroke and vision loss). Some surgeons believe embolisation obscures tumour margins.

Blood supply usually from (branches of) IMAX but can be direct from ICA and can be bilateral.

The histology confirms the pathology. What are the typical features seen?

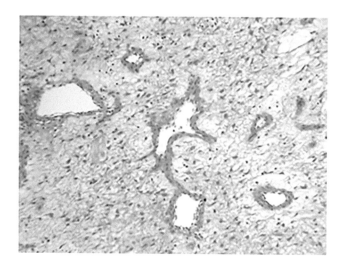

• No capsule
- Irregular vascular component
- High stromal collagen content
- Lack of smooth muscle and elastin

The lack of smooth muscle and elastin is the reason it readily bleeds (vascular constriction is not effective).

The tumour has been resected. What follow-up would you offer?

Dependent on location and access to possible recurrence sites.

Endoscopic surveillance and/or serial imaging is often required but debate exists on time interval between scans.

Recurrence occurs typically at 12–24 months, but spontaneous regression of small residuals has also been observed.

Possible surveillance includes clinical observation with a baseline scan at 4–6 months and serial scans every 12 months.

Laryngomalacia

MATTHEW ELLIS

A 6-month-old boy is referred to outpatient clinic with a 3-month history of increasing noisy breathing occurring episodically, particularly at night and while feeding or upset. He was born at term with an uncomplicated delivery and there was no respiratory distress in the neonatal period. His mother is concerned that he is not feeding well or putting on weight.

What is laryngomalacia?

This is the most common cause of stridor in infants caused by collapse of the supraglottic structures on inspiration. It presents within the first few weeks of life. The symptoms peak at around 6 months of age and usually resolve spontaneously by the end of the second year.

Important elements in the history

- Episodic high-pitched inspiratory stridor
- Stridor worsens while crying or in supine position
- Intermittent cough or choking with feeding
- Recurrent chest infections – although these may also be more suggestive of a laryngeal cleft

Signs of severe laryngomalacia

- Increased work of breathing
- Failure to thrive
- Crossing multiple centiles for body weight
- Tracheal tug
- Sternal recession
- Cyanosis

Laryngomalacia will feature in the differential diagnosis of most cases of noisy breathing in infants. There is a slight male preponderance (1.6:1) and the natural history is of normal breathing at birth, onset of symptoms within the first month, increasing until around 6 months then spontaneously improving by age of 2 years. Conservative management is adequate for 70% of patients. The condition causes difficulty feeding and increased metabolic expenditure on work of breathing so a child putting on weight according to WHO centiles is a reassuring sign.

Investigations

- Flexible nasendoscopy
- Polysomnography
- Echocardiography
- Microlaryngoscopy

The anaesthetic technique used is crucial to attain an adequate view of the vocal cords. A tubeless technique with spontaneous ventilation provides an unobstructed view and may allow evaluation of vocal cord mobility. The technique requires an experienced anaesthetist.

What are the complications of laryngomalacia?

- Feeding difficulties, failure to thrive
- Cor pulmonale
- Pectus excavatum

What are the anatomical features of laryngomalacia?

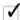
- Shortened aryepiglottic folds
- Omega-shaped retroflexed epiglottis
- Normal vocal cord mobility
- Dynamic collapse of supraglottic structures on inspiration
- Oedema of the posterior glottis

Describe the aetiology of laryngomalacia

The aetiology is poorly understood; two common theories are the neurologic and cartilaginous theories. In the neurologic theory, there is sensorineuromotor dysfunction, reduced neuromuscular tone and laryngeal coordination. Gastroesophageal reflux may contribute to mucosal oedema and reduced laryngeal sensation. Increased work of breathing may in turn exacerbate reflux owing to negative intrathoracic pressure. In the cartilaginous theory, immature laryngeal cartilage offers insufficient mechanical resistance to collapse, causing collapse of the supraglottic structures on inspiration. The resulting mucosal trauma causes oedema, further worsening the stridor. This theory has not been supported by histopathology or the lack of laryngomalacia in premature babies and at birth. The commonest theory is now that laryngomalacia is a normal anatomical variant which is predisposed to collapse on inspiration until such time as the airway grows and the tissues mature.

Laryngomalacia exists on a continuum of airway pathologies with pharyngomalacia above and tracheomalacia and bronchomalacia below.

What are the non-surgical treatment options for laryngomalacia?

- Feeding modification:
- Upright positioning while feeding
- Pacing of feeding
- Frequent burping
- Texture modification with thickener
- Medical treatment of reflux with H2-receptor antagonist and/or proton pump inhibitor

What are the known coexisting comorbidities?

- Gastroesophageal reflux
- Neurologic conditions, Down syndrome
- Cardiac comorbidity

In those that cases that do have an MLB it has been reported that synchronous airway abnormalities can be found in up to a third of cases e.g. tracheomalacia, subglottic stenosis or vocal cord paralysis.

Describe the main steps of a supraglottoplasty

- Preoperative discussion with anaesthetist regarding ventilation technique
- Airway assessment with Benjamin–Lindholm laryngoscope and Hopkins endoscope
- Topical lignocaine to reduce the risk of laryngospasm
- Division of aryepiglottic fold with trimming of arytenoid mucosa in selected cases
- Topical adrenaline if required for bleeding

What are the main complications of supraglottoplasty?

- Early: Bleeding into the airway, airway oedema, infection
- Intermediate: Granulation tissue, aspiration
- Late: Mucosal webbing, supraglottic stenosis

Microtia

SUNIL SHARMA

In the ENT clinic you are asked to see the following patient referred by audiology with the ear abnormality shown below.

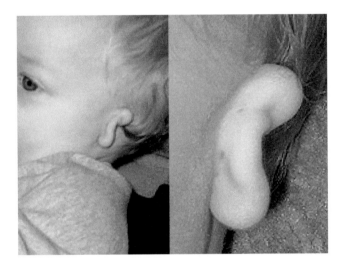

Please describe this image

'This is a clinical photograph of the left ear demonstrating evidence of microtia'.

What is the classification?

There are many classification systems that you will see described in various textbooks (e.g. Marx, Weerda, Meurman, Hunter, Tanzer, Nagata). It is worth being aware of one classification system that you are comfortable with and describing it in the exam if asked. Many microtia surgeons do not use the Marx classification as it has little practical use, but it's worth finding out what your local microtia surgeon uses and reading up on that.

What are the main considerations in managing this child?

- Importance of MDT approach, child should be seen in a dedicated microtia clinic.
- Hearing rehabilitation. 15%–30% have bilateral hearing loss. Implement the use of a softband BC aid as early as possible. By at least the age of 5 a percutaneous BAHA can be considered – increasingly these are being offered for younger children. MEIs are also an option depending on the middle ear and mastoid anatomy. The need for imaging should be directed by the options being considered.

- Psychology.
- Cosmesis: Options here include no surgery, a bone-anchored prosthesis or reconstruction with autologous costal cartilage/alloplastic materials (e.g. Medpor).

When planning positioning for surgical hearing rehabilitation, what is the most important consideration?

It is crucial to position any hearing implant components and incisions an adequate distance from the microtic ear so as not to compromise future reconstruction options.

When would you consider pinna reconstruction, and why?

Reconstruction at around 10 years old will allow the child to be involved in decision making and allow enough costal cartilage to be available if considering autologous costal cartilage.

What syndromes are associated with this condition?

Microtia is only associated with syndromes in around 5% of cases, but can be associated with:

- Treacher Collins syndrome, CHARGE, branchio-oto-renal syndrome, hemifacial microsomias, Nager syndrome, foetal alcohol syndrome, Klippel–Feil syndrome

 Further reading:

UK Care Standards for the Management of Patients with Microtia and Atresia (March 2015). http://www.bapras.org.uk/professionals/clinical-guidance

Obstructive Sleep Apnoea

LAKHBINDER PABLA

You are the consultant in clinic and the next patient is a 3-year-old boy with a history of snoring and his parents are worried about his sleep. On examination, he has large tonsils with no signs of infection. What else would you like to ask the parents?

Important elements in the history

 • Snoring with pauses in breathing/apnoeas
- Restlessness
- Bedwetting/enuresis
- Tiredness, recurrent tonsillitis
- Poor concentration and behaviour
- Poor weight gain
- Mouth breathing
- Nasal symptoms
- Comorbidities (higher incidence of OSA and more likely to be severe):
  - Down syndrome
  - Neuromuscular disease
  - Craniofacial abnormalities
  - Achondroplasia
  - Mucopolysaccharidosis
  - Prader–Willi syndrome

Clinically this patient has OSA. How would you manage this patient?

'I would discuss the diagnosis of OSA and the varying degrees of severity. Depending on the history and the presence of other coexisting conditions, I would discuss the options of watchful waiting, further sleep investigations for risk stratification and surgical options for treatment'.

The examiner wants you to demonstrate an understanding of the spectrum of sleep-disordered breathing and OSA with a logical strategy for risk stratification of these patients. The use of sleep studies for risk stratification in healthy children is controversial as it is not reliable and is a poor predictor of respiratory complications post-surgery.

Options for further management include:

1. Watchful waiting: Most cases resolve by 7–8 years of age, but parents need to be counselled on the pros and cons including the potential neurobehavioral and cognitive effects in some cases of significant OSA.
2. Referral for paediatric sleep investigations to confirm diagnosis or assess severity and aid triage to tertiary-level care.
3. Adenotonsillectomy: Coblation versus cold steel/bipolar.

When would you refer for sleep investigations?

Sleep investigations are not routinely necessary in an otherwise fit and well child with a convincing history of OSA, large tonsils and nasal obstruction on examination in clinic.

Most regional children's hospitals have their own protocol on investigations, which are produced jointly with the local paediatric respiratory team and account for the resources available in that particular department. They are largely based on the UK multidisciplinary working party consensus statement for the indications for referral for paediatric respiratory sleep investigations (2009). These recommendations have recently been updated: 'Safe delivery of paediatric ENT surgery in the UK: A national strategy (2019)'. This update was required due to the increasing number of referrals to specialist centres of children requiring routine ENT surgery.

 Robb PJ, Bew S, Kubba H et al. Tonsillectomy and adenoidectomy in children with sleep-related breathing disorders: Consensus statement of a UK multidisciplinary working party. *Annals of the Royal College of Surgeons of England.* 2009;91(5):371–3.

Refer for paediatric sleep investigations if:

- Diagnosis of OSA is unclear or inconsistent
- Down syndrome
- Cerebral palsy
- Hypotonia or neuromuscular disorders
- Craniofacial anomalies
- Mucopolysaccharidosis
- Obesity
- Significant comorbidity such as congenital heart disease, chronic lung disease
- Residual symptoms after adenotonsillectomy

What is coblation and why is it being used in adenotonsillectomy for paediatric OSA?

'Coblation technology uses radiofrequency energy passed through an isotonic saline solution to create a controlled plasma field which dissociates tissue by breaking ionic intercellular bonds. It works at a lower temperature of around 40–70 degrees Celsius compared to 400–600 degrees Celsius in electrocautery'.

'My preferred technique is intracapsular coblation tonsillotomy because, in addition to the low bleeding risk, it is associated with a lower working temperature and does not breach the capsule of the tonsil which results in lower post-operative pain scores'.

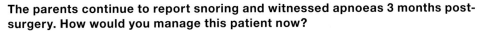

The parents continue to report snoring and witnessed apnoeas 3 months post-surgery. How would you manage this patient now?

- Check the oropharynx and nasopharynx for regrowth/remnants.
- If there is any nasal obstruction/rhinitis, commence a trial of nasal steroid spray.
- Evaluate the presence of any other underlying conditions such as neuromuscular problems, pharyngomalacia and craniofacial abnormalities.
- Repeat the sleep study – is there any residual OSA or central pauses?
- If there are persistent symptoms and an obstructive pattern on sleep investigations, refer to a respiratory paediatrician for a trial of nasal CPAP.

Types of respiratory investigations: Gold standard investigation is an in-hospital, overnight full polysomnogram, which is expensive and time-consuming. Therefore, alternatives are often used.

	Pulse Oximetry	**Respiratory Polygraphy**	**Full Polysomnogram (PSG)**
Advantages	Can be used at home or in hospital Well tolerated Relatively inexpensive Scoring systems for OSA available (e.g. McGill scoring criteria)	Can be used at home or in hospital Can distinguish between central and obstructive pauses Monitors HR, oxygen saturations, thoracic and abdominal excursion, nasal flow, microphone and position sensors	Hospital investigation only Measures everything done by respiratory polygraphy as well as limited EEG, electrooculography, 3-lead ECG and limb leads
Disadvantages	Can't separate central from obstructive problems Variable results from different machines Low sensitivity	More expensive	Most expensive

Further reading:

- Cochrane review of tonsillectomy versus adenotonsillectomy versus non-surgical treatment for OSA.

  Venekamp RP, Hearne BJ, Chandrasekharan D, Blackshaw H, Lim J, Schilder AGM. Tonsillectomy or adenotonsillectomy versus non-surgical management for obstructive sleep-disordered breathing in children. *Cochrane Database of Systematic Reviews* 2015, 10.

- CHAT study: RCT of adenotonsillectomy versus watchful waiting in children aged 5–9 years, primary outcome measure was neurocognitive outcomes, multiple secondary outcomes. Completed and published results.

  Marcus CL, Moore RH, Rosen CL et al. A randomized trial of adenotonsillectomy for childhood sleep apnea. *New England Journal of Medicine.* 2013;368(25):2366–76.

- POSTA Trial: Prospective RCT of adenotonsillectomy versus watchful waiting in children aged 3–5 years. Primary outcome measure intellectual test outcomes. Currently recruiting.

  Waters KA, Chawla J, Harris MA et al. Rationale for and design of the 'POSTA' study: Evaluation of neurocognitive outcomes after immediate adenotonsillectomy compared to watchful waiting in preschool children. *BMC Pediatrics.* 2017;17(1):47.

Otitis Media

ROBERT NASH

Describe this image

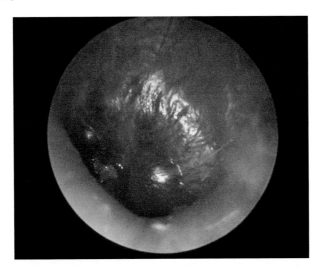

'*This is clinical photograph of an otoendoscopic view of the left TM. There is erythema and injection of a bulging TM in keeping with a diagnosis of acute otitis media (AOM)*'.

What is otitis media?

'*Otitis media describes a range of conditions characterised by inflammation of the middle ear cleft. These can be classified by the timescale and cause of the inflammation*'.

This is a very broad question. There are international societies dedicated to the study of otitis media! It is best to keep things simple. Avoid going into lengthy discussions about all the possible forms of otitis media and the extensive debate about their pathogenesis. There is a range of classification systems, and you cannot be sure which the examiners are looking for. If the examiners want further information, they will ask, and you can give them the information, but it is usually beneficial to move the viva on to the more important questions.

'*In the case of this photograph, the patient has AOM. This describes an acute infection of the middle ear cleft from a bacterial or viral pathogen*'.

By relating the question back to the photograph, you are providing more information in the field they are examining and moving the viva forward in a productive way.

Important elements in the history

- Age of the patient
- Degree to which symptoms are affecting patient – otalgia, hearing loss, otorrhoea
- Symptoms of systemic illness – fever, responsiveness, behaviour
- Symptoms of local complications – facial weakness, dizziness, otalgia, diplopia, neck swelling
- Previous symptoms giving information on underlying cause – pre-existing hearing loss, history of prior infections

Potential complications of acute otitis media

- Mastoiditis
- Facial paresis
- Meningitis
- Suppurative labyrinthitis
- Gradenigo syndrome
- Temporal lobe abscess/empyaema
- Bezold's abscess (abscess deep to SCM)
- Luc's abscess (temporal abscess)
- Citelli's abscess (digastric triangle or occipital region)

Would you prescribe this patient antibiotics?

'I would follow the NICE guidelines for the management of AOM. These recommend withholding antibiotics for 3 days in patients who are not systemically unwell. I would review the situation after 72 hours and provide safety netting advice to return if the patient became less well'.

In a viva such as this, it is arguably prudent to be more interventional, and prescribe antibiotics at an early stage. This can be justified by reminding the examiner that if a patient has been referred to an ENT surgeon, then usually there is sufficient concern to warrant prescription. However, it can be beneficial to quote and follow national guidelines – particularly when they are published by NICE.

 https://www.cochrane.org/CD000219/ARI_antibiotics-for-acute-middle-ear-infection-acute-otitis-media-in-children

Would any features in the history or assessment change your mind?

'Febrile illness in children below the age of 3 months would warrant an immediate admission and paediatric review. Equally, if there were signs or symptoms that made me concerned about the development of a complication of AOM, I would consider immediate admission. If there were signs of systemic upset, persistent otorrhoea, or AOM in a child below 2 years, I would prescribe antibiotics

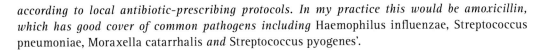

according to local antibiotic-prescribing protocols. In my practice this would be amoxicillin, which has good cover of common pathogens including Haemophilus influenzae, Streptococcus pneumoniae, Moraxella catarrhalis *and* Streptococcus pyogenes'.

Under what circumstances would you consider acute myringotomy?

'*Surgical treatment of AOM is very rarely required. Indications would include persistent symptomatic infection despite adequate antibiotic treatment, signs and symptoms of the development of complications of AOM such as facial weakness, and the need to obtain a specimen of pus for microbiological assessment*'.

If the patient developed mastoiditis how would you proceed?

Common discussion themes include:

- Whether you would perform a CT scan
- Whether you would manage conservatively or surgically
- Whether you would place a grommet at the time of surgery
- How you would manage concomitant lateral sinus thrombosis
- How you would perform a cortical mastoidectomy for an acute mastoiditis

Further reading:

See the NICE clinical knowledge summary on acute otitis media. *https://cks.nice.org.uk/otitis-media-acute#!topicsummary*

Atkinson H, Wallis S, Coatesworth AP. Acute otitis media. *Postgraduate Medicine.* 2015 May;127(4):386–90.

Ren Y, Sethi RKV, Stankovic KM. Acute Otitis Media and Associated Complications in United States Emergency Departments. *Otology and Neurotology.* 2018 Sep;39(8):1005–1011.

If the discussion moves on to OME...

Even though this is a seemingly simple topic you should be prepared on the following areas:

- Tympanometry – An objective measure of TM compliance using reflected sound. Be able to explain the components of a tympanometer and how it works, what the axes of the pressure graph represent, and what the thresholds are for different types of traces.
- Evidence for the management of OME – How you decide between conservative management and grommets using NICE guidelines. Different types of grommets, the role of adenoidectomy and optimisation of nasal function in recurrent disease, the relevance of immune function and your rates of post-grommet complications.
- OME in special cases – Be aware of current guidelines and be able to explain your management strategy for children with Down syndrome, cleft palate, primary ciliary dyskinaesia and children who have had RT.

Paediatric Airway Compromise

LAKHBINDER PABLA

Paediatric airway compromise can come up in a variety of scenarios ranging from newborn infants with bilateral choanal atresia or vocal cord palsies to older children with subglottic stenosis or foreign bodies. This section includes a particular scenario of subglottic stenosis but the presented systematic approach to history, examination and initial assessment of the airway is applicable to many situations and often the area where the examiners are looking for pass/fail marks.

You are on call and in the outpatient clinic. The duty A&E consultant calls you to discuss a 10-year-old girl in paediatric resuscitation with a history of noisy breathing and increased respiratory effort. How would you proceed?

The examiner wants to know that you will make this child a priority as this is a potential airway emergency. Make clear that you would go to see the child immediately, obtain a thorough history and examine in a systematic manner.

Important elements in the history

 • Onset and duration of noisy breathing (sudden – consider foreign body, age of onset is key to predicting potential pathology)
- Recent history of URTI (possible existing stenosis worsened by infection)
- Previous surgery/intubation (subglottic stenosis, vocal cord paresis)
- Cough or choking spells (foreign body)
- Cyanotic spells (tracheal pathology or vascular compression)
- Cry/abnormal voice (vocal cord pathology, papillomas)
- Feeding difficulty and weight gain
- Respiratory problems
- Vaccination history
- Antenatal and birth problems

Examination

'Firstly, I would characterise the noisy breathing to ascertain the likely level of obstruction'.

Distinguish between stertor and stridor.

Site of pathology	Characteristic of noise	Voice
Supralaryngeal/pharynx	Stertor	Muffled
Supraglottis/glottis	Inspiratory stridor	Hoarse
Subglottis	Biphasic stridor	Normal
Trachea/bronchi	Expiratory stridor	Normal

'Furthermore, I would assess the respiratory effort, concentrating on the efficiency and effectiveness of breathing'.

This would include:

- Degree of respiratory effort
  - Tracheal tug (comes first)
  - Sternal and intercostal recession
  - Opisthotonic posture (neck extended)
- Efficacy of breathing: respiratory rate, oxygen saturation
- Chest examination: wheeze, reduced air entry, crackles
- Conscious level/tiredness

Also check for cutaneous haemangiomas and craniofacial abnormalities.

Have a higher index of suspicion for patients with the following:

- Biphasic stridor
- Previous intubation
- Oxygen requirement
- Cyanotic episodes
- Parental and paediatrician concern

This child has had a heart transplant in the past and parents report a recent URTI. She is aware of her surroundings but looks to be working hard with a biphasic stridor and an elevated respiratory rate. What would you do next?

(You may be given an observation chart at this point to highlight these warning signs)

Split the management into immediate management to temporise the situation whilst planning for more definitive management with the appropriate teams:

Immediate: Maintain child's airway and minimise distress

- High-flow oxygen
- Nebulised adrenaline: 1 mL of 1 in 1000 adrenaline made up to 5 mL with normal saline
- Dexamethasone: 0.15–0.6 mg/kg oral or IV
- Contact senior paediatric anaesthetist on call to arrange transfer to theatre for airway assessment and secure the airway if needed
- Contact theatre coordinator to book onto theatre emergency list and advise on equipment needed (include suspension microlaryngoscopy equipment, flexible bronchoscope, age-appropriate Storz ventilating bronchoscope and tracheostomy set)

Definitive management in theatre:

- Inhalational induction
- Vocal cords to be sprayed with topical 4% lidocaine
- Spontaneous ventilation with oxygenation/anaesthetic via a nasopharyngeal airway to maintain anaesthesia
- Unstable airway: Inspect and secure airway/ventilation with:
  - Ventilating bronchoscope
  - Railroad an ETT over a Hopkins rod and introduce into the airway using laryngoscope
  - Tracheostomy if above fails or too unstable to attempt
- If stable, perform microlaryngobronchoscopy with 0° or 30° Hopkins rod and anaesthetic laryngoscope paying particular attention to:
  - Pharynx: Pharyngomalacia, large obstructive tonsils, tongue base, lingual cyst
  - Larynx: Laryngomalacia, vocal cord palsy, webs, respiratory papillomas
  - Subglottis: Stenosis, haemangioma
  - Trachea: Tracheomalacia, tracheoesophageal fistula, pulsatile external compression, granulations, tracheitis
  - Carina/main bronchi: Bronchomalacia, foreign body, granulations/inflammation

In a child with significant micrognathia, attempts at inspection of the airway using a far lateral approach are useful. This involves pushing the tongue with the anaesthetic laryngoscope blade from the right to the left allowing the Hopkins rod or ET tube to enter from the right and towards the larynx.

What are the differences between an adult and paediatric airway?

- Narrow nares
- Large tongue
- Large occiput
- Smaller and more compressible airways
- Larynx positioned higher at C3–C4 (C6 in adults) and more anterior
- Larger, omega-shaped epiglottis
- Subglottis relatively smaller and more reactive

How does a neonatal or paediatric tracheostomy differ from an adult tracheostomy?

- Excise subcutaneous fat
- Vertical slit tracheotomy rather than window cut-out in trachea
- Stoma maturation sutures
- Always have stay sutures in place until first tracheostomy tube change
- Beware that innominate vessels are more likely to be found in the neck

This child has subglottic stenosis exacerbated by inflammation from a recent URTI. Make sure you are aware of the Myer–Cotton classification for paediatric subglottic stenosis.

Myer–Cotton grading system for subglottic stenosis:

Classification of obstruction	From	To
Grade I	0%	50%
Grade II	51%	70%
Grade III	71%	99%
Grade IV	No detectable lumen	

 Read about the management options for subglottic stenosis, including balloon dilatation and laryngotracheal reconstruction in severe cases/failed balloon dilatation.

Paediatric tracheostomy tubes

There are lots of different types of paediatric tracheostomy tubes, some of which are used in special circumstances in specialist units. The GOSH airway sizing chart provides an overview of the types of tracheostomy tubes available according to age as well as a very useful guide on ventilating bronchoscope and ET tube sizes. You are not expected to know the details of every type of tracheostomy tube in the chart but familiarise yourself with the most commonly used tubes described next.

- Bivona:
  - Most commonly used
  - Comes as two main types: Neonatal (largest size 4.0) and paediatric tracheostomy tubes (go up to size 5.5)
  - Paediatric tubes – standard length; neonatal tubes – shorter lengths
  - Cuffed or non-cuffed available
  - Caution: Check with local department if compatible with MRI
  - Variations include flextend and hyperflex Bivona tubes
- Shiley:
  - Three main types: Neonatal (largest size 4.5), paediatric standard length tracheostomy tubes (go up to 6.5) and paediatric longer length tube
  - Cuffed and non-cuffed available
- Tight to shaft:
  - Has a high-pressure low-volume cuff, filled with water rather than air
  - Sometimes used to achieve effective ventilation

GOSH Paediatric Airway Sizing Chart:

Great Ormond Street Hospital Chart for Paediatric Airways

		Preterm–1 month	1–6 months	6–18 months	18 mths –3 yrs	3–6 years	6–9 years	9–13 years	12–14 years
Trachea (transverse diameter mm)		5	5-6	6-7	7-8	8-9	9-10	10-13	13
Great Ormond Street	ID (mm)	3.0	3.5	4.0	4.5	5.0	5.5	6.0	7.0
	OD (mm)	4.5	5.0	6.0	6.7	7.5	8.0	8.7	10.7
Shiley	Size	3.0	3.5	4.0	4.5	5.0	5.5	6.0	6.5
	ID (mm)	3.0	3.5	4.0	4.5	5.0	5.5	6.0	6.5
	OD (mm)	4.5	5.2	5.9	6.5	7.1	7.7	8.3	9.0
	Length (mm) Neonatal		30	32	34	36			
*Cuffed tube available	Paediatric		39	40	41*	42*	44*	46*	
	Long paediatric					50*	52*	54*	56*
Portex (Blue Line)	ID (mm)	3.0	3.5	4.0	4.5	5.0	5.0	6.0	7.0
	OD (mm)	4.2	4.9	5.5	6.2	6.9	6.9	8.3	9.7
Portex (555)	Size		2.5	3.0	3.5	4.0	4.5	5.0	5.5
	ID (mm)		2.5	3.0	3.5	4.0	4.5	5.0	5.5
	OD (mm)		4.5	5.2	5.8	6.5	7.1	7.7	8.3
	Length Neonatal		30	32	34	36			
	Paediatric		30	36	40	44	48	50	52
Bivona	Size	2.5	3.0	3.5	4.0	4.5	5.0	5.5	
All sizes available with Fome Cuff, Aire Cuff and TTS Cuff	ID (mm)	2.5	3.0	3.5	4.0	4.5	5.0	5.5	
	OD (mm)	4.0	4.7	5.3	6.0	6.7	7.3	8.0	
	Length Neonatal		30	32	34	36			
	Paediatric	38	39	40	41	42	44	46	
Bivona Hyperflex	ID (mm)	2.5	3.0	3.5	4.0	4.5	5.0	5.5	
	Usable length (mm)	55	60	65	70	75	80	85	
Bivona Flextend	ID (mm)	2.5	3.0	3.5	4.0	4.5	5.0	5.5	
	Shaft length (mm)	38	39	40	41	42	44	46	
	Flextend length (mm)	10	10	15	15	17.5	20	20	
TracoeMini	ID (mm)	2.5	3.0	3.5	4.0	4.5	5.0	5.5	6.0
	OD (mm)	3.6	4.3	5.0	5.6	6.3	7.0	7.6	8.4
	Length (mm) Neonatal (350)		30	32	34	36			
	Paediatric (355)	32	36	40	44	48	50	55	62
Alder Hey	FG		12-14	16	18	20	22	24	
Negus	FG		16	18	20	22	24	26	28
Chevalier Jackson	FG	14	16	18	20	22	24	26	28
Sheffield	FG		12-14	16	18	20	22	24	26
	ID (mm)		2.9-3.6	4.2	4.9	6.0	6.3	7.0	7.6
Cricoid (AP diameter)	ID (mm)	3.6-4.8	4.8-5.8	5.8-6.5	6.5-7.4	7.4-8.2	8.2-9.0	9.0-10.7	10.7
Bronchoscope (Storz)	Size	2.5	3.0	3.5	4.0	4.5	5.0	6.0	6.0
	ID (mm)	3.5	4.3	5.0	6.0	6.6	7.1	7.5	7.5
	OD (mm)	4.2	5.0	5.7	6.7	7.3	7.8	8.2	8.2
Endotracheal tube (Portex)	ID (mm)	2.5	3.0	3.5	4.0	4.5	5.0	6.0	7.0 8.0
	OD (mm)	3.4	4.2	4.8	5.4	6.2	6.8	8.2	9.6 10.8

(Left-margin group labels: Plastic; Silver)

Table reproduced from *Choosing a paediatric tracheostomy: an update on current practice* DJ Tweedie, CJ Skilbeck, LA Cochrane, J Cooke, ME Wyatt. The Journal of Laryngology & Otology. 2007

Decannulation protocol for paediatric tracheostomy patients

Indications for decannulation:

- Original airway issue resolved or improved enough to attempt decannulation
- No oxygen requirement
- No current or recent upper respiratory chest infection
- Recent microlaryngobronchoscopy to assess suitability for decannulation

Most paediatric departments will have their own version of a decannulation protocol which is broadly based on the following protocol:

Day 1: Admit and downsize tracheostomy tube to size 3.0

Day 2: Cap tracheostomy during daytime hours. If tolerates well, remain capped overnight

Day 3: Remove tracheostomy tube, airtight dressing applied over stoma and observe on ward

Day 4: Able to leave ward but remain in hospital

Day 5: Home

Paediatric Hearing Loss

ROBERT NASH AND JOSEPH MANJALY

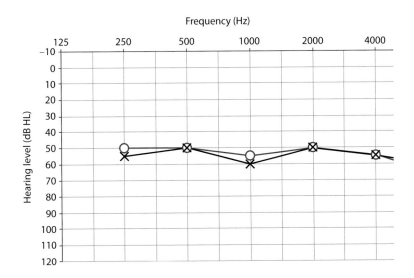

'*This is a pure tone audiogram showing air conduction thresholds of 50–60 dB in the left and the right ear. BC thresholds have not been recorded. This would be consistent with a moderate hearing loss*'.

This child is 24 months old. How do you think this hearing test has been performed?

Age-appropriate audiology is an important topic to revise. A 24-month-old developmentally normal child would typically be tested using play audiometry. It is important to be aware of the ages at which a developmentally normal child would be likely to condition for visual reinforcement, play and pure tone audiometry (see the chapter on Developmental milestones, hearing and speech, autism within this section of the book). Furthermore, it is important to be aware of the options for testing children who cannot be conditioned for behavioural hearing testing. These include tests that are straightforward to perform, such as otoacoustic emissions (OAE), or tests such as tympanograms that do not test hearing, but are surrogate measures which can give more useful clinical information. It is also important to be able to interpret audiograms – in particular, paediatric audiograms that may use measures such as sound field testing (where the child will not cooperate with the use of headphones). See the end of this section for some helpful information.

Important elements in the history

☑ • Age of the patient
- Speech development
- History of ear infections, otorrhoea, otalgia
- History of tugging at the ear
- Family history of hearing loss at a young age
- Comorbidity

On examination, there are dull TMs on both sides, and a tympanogram shows type-B traces in both ears. How would you proceed?

'*These findings suggest a likely diagnosis of bilateral OME. I would follow the NICE guidelines for the management of chronic otitis media (NICE CG60). As this is the first time glue ear has been identified a period of observation is warranted. I would advise on behavioural and educational strategies to minimise the effect of the hearing loss. A 2-year-old child is unlikely to cooperate with autoinflation, but it could be considered in older children. I would review the child in 3 months*'.

At 3 months the patient has a similar hearing loss. You have concerns about speech development. How would you proceed?

You will need to discuss the options with the parents. This hearing loss meets NICE CG60 core criteria for intervention (25–30 dB or worse loss averaged at 0.5–4 kHz in the better ear sustained for at least 3 months). Surgical management in the form of grommet insertion should be considered. Alternatively, hearing aids are an option. If you do proceed with grommet insertion, you should describe the operative technique and the perioperative care, including the follow-up plan.

On review 4 weeks after grommet insertion, repeated audiometry shows a persistent 50 dB hearing loss. How would you proceed?

You should be familiar with the causes of hearing loss. It is possible that the grommets have extruded and the glue has recurred. Examination should reveal this and most of the other causes of conductive hearing loss. It is also possible that the middle ear effusion was a distraction and the patient has an underlying SNHL. Fitting of hearing aids should be considered at an early stage and referral for aetiological investigation should be considered. You should be familiar with the causes of hearing loss and their clinical features. A basic understanding of hearing aid fitting and the types of hearing aids available is important. It is also important to consider that breaking the news of a persistent hearing loss to parents involves good communication skills.

A summary of possible causes of hearing loss in children:

- Conductive
  - Glue ear
  - TM retraction
  - TM perforation
  - Cholesteatoma
  - Congenital or acquired ossicular discontinuity

- Sensorineural
  - Genetic
    - Non-syndromic (70%)
      - Autosomal recessive (75%) (commonest = connexin 26 variants)
      - Autosomal dominant (23%)
      - X-linked (1%)
      - Mitochondrial (1%)
    - As part of a syndrome (30%)
      - Chromosomal – Down, Turner and Patau syndromes
      - Autosomal recessive – Usher, Pendred, Jervell and Lange-Nielsen, osteogenesis imperfecta (less common than dominant inheritance), Waardenburg type 2D, Stickler type 4–5
      - Autosomal dominant – Waardenburg (types 1–4), branchio-oto-renal, Treacher Collins (TCOF1 - 2 dominant, TCOF3 is recessive), NFII, Stickler type 1–3, Crouzon, Apert, osteogenesis imperfecta, osteopetrosis, 22q11 deletion syndrome
      - X-linked – Alport, otopalatodigital syndrome
      - Mitochondrial
  - Environmental
    - Intrauterine infection
      - Toxoplasmosis, rubella, CMV, herpes, HIV, syphilis
    - Alcohol, smoking
    - Ototoxic drugs
    - Ex-prem, SCBU, hypoxia, hyperbilirubinaemia
    - Maternal diabetes and hypothyroidism
    - Idiopathic

A summary of paediatric hearing screening in the UK:

- The NHSP was set up in 2005. It aims to identify children with >40 dB congenital hearing loss in the better ear.
- There are two screening pathways:
  - Well baby pathway (<4 weeks but not before 34 weeks' gestation)
    - Up to two attempts at transient OAE testing, usually before leaving hospital after birth
    - Pass + no risk factors → discharge
    - Pass but risk factors → refer to audiology
    - Fail → AABR → Pass + no risk factors → discharge

        → Fail or risk factors → refer to audiology
    - Risk factors:
      - Parental/professional concern
      - High risk of chronic middle ear problems e.g. Down syndrome, cleft lip/palate

- Craniofacial abnormalities
- Family history of early SNHL
- NICU/SCBU IPPV or ECMO
- Jaundice/hyperbilirubinaemia
- TORCH infection
- Neurodevelopmental condition
- Ototoxic drugs
  - ○ NICU/SCBU pathway
    - One OAE attempt both ears + AABR within 4 weeks corrected age
    - Overall <5% fail screening, of which 1/10 have permanent SNHL

Here is a summary of the objective and subjective age-appropriate ways of assessing children's hearing that you should be familiar with:

- Objective tests
  - ○ Transient OAEs
    - A test of the three rows of OHCs on the basilar membrane
    - Probe to ear canal, series of broadband clicks
    - Stimulus + returned sounds are recorded by microphone → average and frequency analysis
    - Different frequencies tested at different amplitudes
    - Need 3/5 signal-to-noise ratio passes to pass overall
    - Pros: easy to perform, affordable, 97% sensitivity
    - Cons: low specificity, affected by OME and ear canal debris, background noise
    - Note – other types of OAEs exist
      - Spontaneous OAEs
      - Distortion product OAEs
        - ○ Stimulate cochlea with two tones of differing frequency
        - ○ More frequency specific but less sensitive to detecting hearing loss
  - ○ AABR
    - Multiple peak waveform, recalled using the mnemonic 'ECOLI' (eighth nerve, cochlear nucleus, superior olive, lateral lemniscus, inferior colliculus)
    - Multiple frequencies and thresholds
    - Performed asleep or GA
    - Electrode on vertex and test ear mastoid
    - Cons: resource intensive
- Subjective tests
  - ○ Behavioural observation testing
    - Looking for timely changes in facial expression, eyes, head turn and changes in suckling

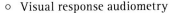

- o Visual response audiometry
  - >6 months old
  - Two testers, parent involved
  - Head-turning to sound→visual reward
  - Frequency and amplitude then varied
- o McCormick toy test
  - >2 years old
  - Paired monosyllabic words familiar to children
- o Play audiometry
  - >20 months–5 years
  - Conditioned test, child asked to perform simple repetitive tasks when tester says go
  - Once conditioned, sounds are played left and right at different frequencies and amplitudes
- o Pure tone audiogram
  - >5 years
  - Affected by motivation and background noise

Further reading:

British Society of Audiology: Recommended procedure for pure-tone air-conduction and bone-conduction threshold audiometry with and without masking, http://www.thebsa.org.uk/wp-content/uploads/2014/04/BSA_RP_PTA_FINAL_24Sept11_MinorAmend06Feb12.pdf

NICE: OME in under 12s: surgery, https://www.nice.org.uk/guidance/cg60

Guidelines for aetiological investigation into mild to moderate bilateral permanent childhood hearing impairment, *https://www.baap.org.uk/uploads/1/1/9/7/119752718/guidelines_for_aetiological_investigation_into_mild_to_moderatebilateral_permanent_childhood_hearing_impairment.pdf*

Periorbital Cellulitis

GARETH LLOYD

This topic can come up in paediatrics or rhinology and is a classic emergency scenario. You must be prepared to answer this in significant detail as the examiner will have high expectations. It is also an opportunity for you to score a high mark.

You are shown a photograph of a child with significant swelling around the right eye involving the upper and lower lids. How would you approach this case?

'In my history I would enquire about the duration of swelling, associated coryzal symptoms and visual disturbance. I would like to examine the nose, eyes and orbits with particular regard to proptosis, visual acuity, colour vision and eye movements for which I would arrange an urgent ophthalmology review'.

How does infection spread from the nose to the periorbital structures?

Typically, there is direct extension of acute sinonasal infection from the ethmoids through the lamina papyracea but spread may be haematological through valveless veins and thrombophlebitis. A small number of children may have a congenital dehiscence or a history of previous facial trauma.

Remember, the frontal and sphenoid sinuses do not develop until 7–12 years old, therefore the maxillary and ethmoid sinus are overwhelmingly the predominant sites of origin.

What are the common organisms?

These are the same bacteria that cause rhinosinusitis:

Streptococcus pneumonia, Haemophilus influenza, Moraxella catarrhalis, Staphylococcus aureus, Streptococcus milleri

Streptococcus milleri tends to be associated with aggressive infections that may extend intracranially.

Fungal infections (e.g. Aspergillus, Rhizopus, Mucor) are rarer in children than in adults.

What are the indications for imaging?

 • Suspicion of intracranial involvement
- Inability to examine eye or open the eyelids
- Eye signs: proptosis, restriction or pain on eye movement, chemosis, relative afferent pupillary defect (RAPD), reduced visual acuity/colour vision/visual field, optic nerve swelling
- Failure to improve or continued pyrexia after 36–48 hours IV antibiotics

How do you assess for RAPD? Why are you assessing colour vision?

It is essential to check for compressive optic neuropathy. A relative afferent papillary defect (Marcus Gunn pupil) is detected with the 'swinging flashlight' test.

A small amount of papillary dilatation when the light is moved from the normal eye to the abnormal eye suggests failure to transmit impulses properly along the optic nerve. This requires immediate confirmation with ophthalmology and is an indication for surgical intervention.

Colour vision should be assessed using Ishihara colour plates or other age-appropriate colour vision tests. Loss of colour vision, specifically the perception of red, is an early sign of optic nerve injury.

What is the ENT UK guidance for medical treatment of paediatric periorbital cellulitis?

• Disease limited to pre-septal cellulitis	**Oral co-amoxiclav** Allergy: Clindamycin
• Clinical suspicion of post-septal cellulitis • Pyrexia • Immunocompromised • Failure to respond to 36–48 hours of oral antibiotics	**IV co-amoxiclav** Mild allergy: IV cefuroxime and metronidazole Severe allergy: Discuss with microbiology Immunocompromised: Discuss with microbiology
• Adjunctive medical management	**Nasal xylometazoline 0.05% (paediatric otrivine)** **Nasal steroids**
• MDT management	**Eye and neuro-observations** – 4 hourly **Urgent ophthalmology** assessment and daily review **Urgent otolaryngology** assessment and daily review

Source: Adapted from Ball S, Okonkwo A, Powell S, Carrie S. Orbital cellulitis management guideline – For adults & paeds, 2017, ENT, UK.

Note that the IV antimicrobial therapy recommended for adults is IV Tazocin (allergy: IV clindamycin and IV ciprofloxacin). Individual units may have their own alternative recommendations based on local microbiology evidence which you may also reference.

What imaging would you arrange?

A contrast-enhanced CT of the orbits, sinuses and brain.

An MRI may also be indicated if frontal cerebritis, abscess or thrombosis of the intracranial sinuses is suspected, or the CT is equivocal. This would typically be second line and follow a discussion with neurosurgery and radiology.

Do you know of a classification scheme for this problem?

The **Chandler classification** is set out as follows with expected clinical findings and rationale for surgical intervention.

It is important to note that the classification does not describe intracranial complications of acute sinusitis (including meningitis and extradural, subdural or intracerebral abscesses) or Pott's puffy tumour.

1. Pre-septal cellulitis	**Infection anterior to the orbital septum** Oedema of the eyelids without visual loss, chemosis or impaired ocular mobility	Medical management only
2. Orbital cellulitis	**Infection posterior to the orbital septum** Diffuse oedema of the peri-ocular adipose tissue Chemosis, proptosis, RAPD, may have mildly limited ocular movement and visual changes	Consider surgery if not improving in 36 hours
3. Sub-periosteal abscess	**Pus collection between bone and periosteum** Chemosis, globe displacement, restricted ocular movement, proptosis and impaired vision	Immediate surgery or consider trial of 24-hour medical management if small abscess without visual compromise in a young child
4. Orbital abscess	**Pus collection within the orbit** Proptosis, severe globe displacement, marked reduced movements and visual loss	Immediate surgery
5. Cavernous sinus thrombosis	**Mural thrombus which may propagate centrally** Picket fence fevers, toxic patient, paralysis of eye (CNIII, IV, VI), facial/corneal numbness (CNV1, V2), proptosis, visual loss. May suddenly become bilateral. May spread to other dural sinuses	Surgery as soon as patient is stable and prior to commencing anticoagulation if used (controversial)

Does a sub-periosteal abscess always need to be drained?

Surgical drainage via an open or endoscopic approach is typically advocated for the treatment of a sub-periosteal abscess; however, these interventions each carry risks. There is a growing body of evidence to suggest that small abscesses in younger children who do not display visual compromise may be safely and successfully treated with medical management.

'These patients must have maximal medical therapy with intravenous antibiotics and adjunctive intranasal decongestants with strict eye and neurological review as per ENT-UK guidelines. If there is any deterioration or a lack of improvement after 24 hours I would have a low threshold for surgical drainage'.

 Useful papers:

Ball S, Okonkwo A, Powell S, Carrie S. Orbital cellulitis management guideline – for adults & paeds. ENT-UK (2017)

Wong SJ, Levi J. Management of pediatric orbital cellulitis: A systematic review. *International Journal of Pediatric Otorhinolaryngology*. 2018 Jul;110:123–9. This paper suggests that if there is no visual compromise, age <9 years old and <3.8 mL abscess volume, then non-surgical management is appropriate.

Recurrent Respiratory Papillomatosis

LAKHBINDER PABLA

You are asked to see a 5-year-old boy with a history of a progressively hoarse voice and no other known comorbidities. What is your differential diagnosis?

 • Chronic laryngitis
- Vocal cord nodules
- Laryngeal papillomas

Common things are common, so don't forget chronic laryngitis possibly due to reflux and vocal cord nodules from shouting at the playground as differentials for a hoarse voice in a child!

You perform a flexible nasendoscopy in clinic and this is what you see:

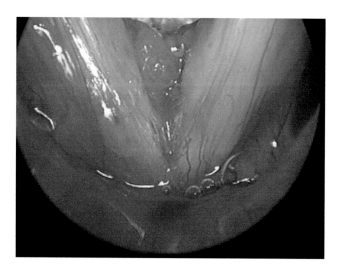

Please describe what you see and how you would manage this case

'This clinical photograph shows multiple laryngeal papillomas involving both vocal cords, particularly the anterior commissure. There is no obvious subglottic extension but this must be considered. I would discuss the likely diagnosis of RRP with the parents and list the patient for a microlaryngobronchoscopy and biopsy to confirm the diagnosis'.

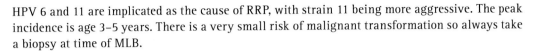

HPV 6 and 11 are implicated as the cause of RRP, with strain 11 being more aggressive. The peak incidence is age 3–5 years. There is a very small risk of malignant transformation so always take a biopsy at time of MLB.

Risk factors for RRP:

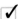 Earlier age of onset (most sensitive predictor of worse prognosis)

HPV 11 (worse prognosis)

Maternal genital warts during pregnancy

Laryngopharyngeal reflux

What treatment options are there for this condition?

'The aim of treatment is to improve the airway whilst ensuring minimal trauma to the laryngeal mucosa in order to preserve the voice. Often multiple procedures are required and management can be divided into medical and surgical options. My preferred approach is surgical microdebridement in the first instance'.

1. Surgical options:
   - *Microdebrider*: Preferred option. Laryngeal microdebrider with a 2.9 mm skimmer blade debrides more accurately and suctions tissue away immediately
   - *Cold steel*: Cupped forceps and scissors with topical 1 in 10,000 adrenaline-soaked neuropatties for haemostasis
   - *CO₂ laser*: Defocussed beam allows precise removal with minimal bleeding; risk of thermal damage to surrounding normal laryngeal mucosa
2. **Surgery and adjuvant medical treatment**: Indicated if multiple surgical procedures every year (>4/year)
3. Adjuvant medical treatment includes:
   - *Gardasil*: Quadrivalent vaccine targeting L1 surface protein on HPV 6, 11, 16 and 18. Given as three courses of intramuscular injection.
   - *Cidofovir*: A cytosine nucleoside analogue that works by inhibiting viral DNA polymerase to prevent HPV DNA synthesis. Estimated 60% cure rate after long course of injections directly into papilomas.
   - *Alpha-Interferon*: Administered systemically and requires regular blood test monitoring due to side effects of bone marrow suppression and hepatitis. Outcomes – 1/3 cured, 1/3 partially better, 1/3 no better. Less commonly used.

 Read up on the HPV vaccination programme (Cervarix bivalent vaccine from 2008 and Gardasil used since 2012). Gardasil vaccination in teenage boys is a political topic.

The most commonly used staging system for RRP is the Derkay score. It is based on a clinical and anatomical score and used to assess the extent of papillomas and predict intervals between surgical intervention. Minimum score = 0, maximum score = 75.

 Derkay CS, Malis DJ, Zalzal G et al. A staging system for assessing severity of disease and response to therapy in recurrent respiratory papillomatosis. *Laryngoscope* 1998;108:935–7.

Syndromes in ENT

SUNIL SHARMA

In the ENT clinic you are asked to see the following child:

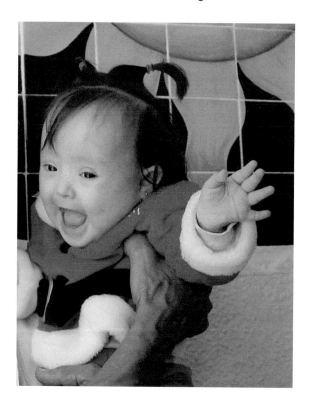

What is the most likely diagnosis? How common is this condition?

'This is a clinical photograph of a child with facial features consistent with a diagnosis of Trisomy 21/Down syndrome. It occurs in 1 in 1000 births per year'.

There are a number of syndromes which commonly feature ENT-related abnormalities. You should aim to recognise many of them from photographs and be able to explain some abnormalities but the condition you must absolutely be prepared for is Down syndrome.

What are the ENT manifestations of this condition?

Have a structured approach for this. In terms of ENT manifestations, divide this into sections:

Otological manifestations:

- Small, low-set ears
- Narrow ear canals
- Vestibular and ossicular abnormalities
- Increased risk of OME (due to palate and skull base anatomy) and lasts for longer, therefore NICE recommends hearing aids first – three reasons: Grommets technically more challenging, often mixed hearing loss therefore will still require hearing aids and repeated grommet insertions likely to be required
- Higher risk of cholesteatoma due to poor Eustachian tube function

Head and neck/airway considerations:

- Adenotonsillar hypertrophy (note atlanto-axial instability, don't require pre-op cervical X-ray unless clinical suspicion of problems)
- Pharyngeal hypotonia
- Macroglossia
- Subglottic stenosis (congenital and acquired due to cardiac surgery)
- Higher risk of tracheobronchomalacia
- Higher risk of sinonasal disease
- Hypothyroidism

What facial features are associated with this condition?

- Brachycephaly
- Upslanting palpebral fissures
- Epicanthic folds
- Hypertelorism
- Low nasal bridge, small nose

What other features are associated with this condition?

- Patent ductus arteriosus (cardiac surgery means greater risk of vocal fold palsy)
- Situs inversus
- VSD/ASD

Read NICE guidelines for management of OME (CG60).

Make sure you revise the following syndromes and familiarise yourself with classic features from looking at photos online, such that you can make a diagnosis quickly in a viva or clinical station:

Treacher Collins syndrome

- Incidence 1:10,000
- First branchial arch anomaly, autosomal dominant or recessive, variable expression, TCOF 1-3 loci
- Down-slanting palpebral fissures
- Maxillary hypoplasia
- Cleft palate
- Telecanthus
- Prominent nose, flat malar, broad mouth
- Airway management options include nasopharyngeal airway, tracheostomy, mandibular distraction aged 3–4 years

Otological considerations:

- Microtia and atresia, auricular tags and pits
- Higher risk of OME
- Ossicular abnormalities
- Cochlear, vestibular aqueduct and facial nerve abnormalities in some cases
- Hearing rehabilitation via BC aids

Goldenhar syndrome

- Hemifacial microsomia
- First and second branchial arch anomalies
- Vertebral anomalies
- Inner, middle and external ear abnormalities
- Absent facial nerve
- Maxillary/mandibular hypoplasia
- Epibulbar dermoids
- Renal and cardiac abnormalities

Pierre Robin sequence

- Micrognathia, leads to relative macroglossia/glossoptosis, leads to inhibited cleft fusion, leading to cleft palate
- Management is with a nasopharyngeal airway, CPAP and, rarely, tracheostomy

Craniosynostoses

Crouzon syndrome:

- *FGFR2* gene related
- Premature fusion of cranial sutures
- Midface hypoplasia, hypertelorism, exorbitism
- OME and ossicular abnormalities, EAC atresia, high-riding jugular bulb
- OSA, high-arched palate
- Narrow PNS, choanal atresia sometimes
- Relative septal overgrowth
- Prognathic jaw
- Depressed nasal bridge

Apert syndrome:

- Similar to Crouzon, but finger abnormalities (syndactyly) and increased risk of learning difficulties

Management is:

- Craniofacial surgery
- Neurosurgery to control cerebrospinal fluid pressure
- Adenotonsillectomy for OSA
- Grommets for OME
- Airway management is with nasopharyngeal airway, CPAP and tracheostomy (note 'shield' trachea)

Velo-cardio-facial syndrome

- Also known as DiGeorge syndrome, 22q11 deletion
- 1:2000, autosomal dominant
- Makes up 5%–8% of all cleft palates
- 20% have Pierre Robin sequence
- Hypoparathyroidism and absent thymus
- Long hypotonic flaccid facies, prominent nasal bridge, narrow nasal cavity, retrognathia
- Medialised ICA (beware in adenoidectomy)
- Laryngeal webs and laryngomalacia
- Microtia, OME and SNHL
- Cardiac disorders, skeletal disorders and learning difficulties

Mucopolysaccharidoses

- OSA
- Short neck, abnormal cervical vertebrae

- High epiglottis, narrow nasopharynx, mandibular hypoplasia
- Adenotonsillar hypertrophy and macroglossia
- Abnormal tracheobronchial cartilage
- Management is with adenotonsillectomy (doesn't always help, CPAP, tongue reduction surgery and tracheostomy)

Achondroplasia

- OSA and central sleep apnoea, therefore a sleep study is essential

Thyroglossal Duct Cyst

JESSICA BEWICK

This is a straightforward scenario which you should be aiming to score highly on.

A 3-year-old child is referred by their GP with a midline neck lump. It has been present for 6 months and is asymptomatic but mum is worried it is cancer. How would you approach this in clinic?

Malignancy in a child with a midline neck lump is exceptionally rare. With the 6-month history you can be relatively confident in reassuring mum early on in the consultation that this is unlikely to be a malignant process.

Important areas in the history and examination

- Associated infections
- Fluctuation in size
- Skin changes
- Associated neck lumps
- Other congenital anomalies
- PMH in relation to birth history and previous anaesthetics

'When examining the child, I would specifically be looking to see if the lump moves on swallowing and tongue protrusion along with the site of the lump itself'.

There is a 2-cm cystic-feeling mass in the lower neck at the level of the cricoid with normal overlying skin and no signs or history of previous infection; it moves on swallowing and tongue protrusion. The child is otherwise well. What would your next step be?

'Clinically this would be most in keeping with a thyroglossal duct cyst although the differential includes a dermoid and within this region of the neck a lesion of the thyroid isthmus. I would arrange an ultrasound to confirm cystic nature of the lump and the presence of an anatomically normal thyroid gland (as it is possible that a thyroglossal cyst contains the only functional thyroid tissue). I would counsel the parents that most likely the treatment will be surgical'.

The scan strongly suggests a thyroglossal duct cyst with normal thyroid. Can you outline your surgical technique for removing thyroglossal duct cysts?

In the appropriately anaesthetised and intubated patient*, extended Sistrunk procedure:

- Position with neck roll and head ring
- Healthy skin: Neck crease incision, in this case, level inferior border of the lump with enough access to explore thyroid isthmus and up to the tongue base**
- Unhealthy skin: Excise previous infective tissue, being careful to take normal tissue around the cyst
- Wide local en bloc excision*** dissecting the medial 1/3 of the strap muscles from the level of the thyroid isthmus up to the central portion of the hyoid bone then removing a core of tissue en bloc up towards the tongue base and foramen caecum (using bimanual palpation to guide if required).
- Closure of the tongue base, strap muscles help with haemostasis and cosmesis
- Insert a drain as these tend to ooze

*Could you do this with an LMA rather than an ETT? No, it is possible one may need to bimanually palpate the tongue base and manipulate the neck during surgery, hence an LMA would be obstructive and unsafe in this instance.

**In reality these are often done in a small child with a short neck, hence an incision midway between the hyoid and cricoid is adequate.

***Why a wide local incision? Thyroglossal tracts usually have extensive arborisation at all levels (the Christmas tree analogy) and by dissecting straight onto the tract there is a significant risk of recurrence.

The child's parents want to know why such a small lump which isn't cancer needs such an extensive procedure.

'I would explain (using diagrams to explain the embryological development if helpful) that removing just the lump carries almost 100% risk of recurrence. Removing the cyst and central hyoid reduces this to 50% and following up to the tongue base further reduces the rate to 5%–6% (classic Sistrunk procedure). Extending this to the thyroid isthmus is thought to reduce the risk of recurrence to 2%–3%'.

You, as the consultant, have had a busy morning clinic which has overrun. Your registrar had helpfully gotten the patient ready for theatre and has already started raising skin flaps when you arrive. You scrub in and while asking the registrar to describe the embryological development of the thyroid gland it becomes apparent that the USS performed previously does not mention the presence of a thyroid gland. What would you do?

Point out that this is an avoidable situation and that by planning theatre lists adequately this should not happen. But in this instance you might:

- Contact the radiologist who performed the scan to comment further on the image.
- If unable to comment, ask for an urgent on-the-table ultrasound of the neck.
- Another option is to explore down to the thyroid gland to confirm its presence.

Neither you nor the radiologist can locate a normal thyroid. What would you do?

'I would ask for the parents to be brought to the theatre suite and ask the theatre sister in charge/ manager to accompany me in a private room to discuss with the parents what has happened and what my concern is (that the child will need lifelong thyroid replacement). Personally, I would want to proceed with the operation to remove the tract which has a risk of future infection and malignancy. I would contact the on-call paediatric consultant +/– endocrinologist if required to make the appropriate plan for the patient post-operatively. I would meet again with the parents following the procedure and apologise for what has happened, discuss the case in a future departmental morbidity and mortality meeting and fill out an incident form'.

Further reading:

Pelausa ME, Forte V. Sistrunk revisited: A 10-year review of revision thyroglossal duct surgery at Toronto's Hospital for Sick Children. *The Journal of Otolaryngology*, 1989;18(7):325–33.

Sistrunk WE. The surgical treatment of cysts of the thyroglossal tract. *Annals of Surgery*, 1920;71(2):121.

Ubayasiri KM, Brocklehurst J, Judd O, Beasley N. A decade of experience of thyroglossal cyst excision. *Annals of the Royal College of Surgeons of England*, 2013;95(4):263–5.

Ahmed J, Leong A, Jonas N, Grainger J, Hartley B. The extended Sistrunk procedure for the management of thyroglossal duct cysts in children: How we do it. *Clinical Otolaryngology*, 2011;36:271–5.

Tonsillitis and Post-Tonsillectomy Bleeding

GARETH LLOYD

This is a topic that you must know thoroughly. You can refer to your local CCG policies where appropriate but avoid turning a clinical scenario into a political one.

 Check the latest national guidelines for indications for tonsil surgery and relevant ENT-UK position papers as these may change.

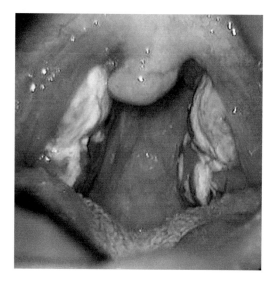

Image Credit: Welleschik • CC BY-SA 3.0. https://commons.wikimedia.org/

'*This is a clinical photograph of the oropharynx displaying Brodsky grade 2 tonsils with bilateral exudate. This is in keeping with acute bacterial tonsillitis but may represent infectious mononucleosis. I would like to take a full history to explore the patient's symptoms and comorbidity, including the severity and duration of this problem. I would perform a full head and neck examination with additional abdominal examination if I am suspicious of glandular fever*'.

Why do we have tonsils?

The palatine tonsils form part of Waldeyer's ring of lymphoid tissue along with the adenoids and lingual tonsil. They function to sample air- and foodborne antigens for the immune system, important in activating and proliferating B cells.

What common pathogens cause tonsillitis?

Viral infections are most common, typically adenovirus which is self-limiting. EBV is associated with infectious mononucleosis (glandular fever) and may resemble Streptococcal infection. Other viruses include Coxsackie-A, parainfluenza, CMV and RSV.

The main bacterial cause is GABHS but consider diphtheria if adherent membranes present and anaerobes such as *Bacteroides* or *Fusobacterium necrophorum* are present.

Viral	Adenovirus EBV Enteroviruses (Coxsackie-A, Rhinovirus) Influenza, parainfluenza CMV *Chlamydia trachomatis*
Bacterial	Group A/B/C/G streptococci *Corynebacterium diphtheriae* *Bacteroides* species *Fusobacterium* species
Mycoplasma	*Mycoplasma pneumoniae*
Fungi	*Candida* species
Parasites	*Toxoplasma gondii*

What is the treatment for tonsillitis?

Viral tonsillitis is self-limiting. Antibiotics should be avoided and patients advised to use analgesia, nonsteroidal anti-inflammatory drugs and drink adequate fluids. NICE guidelines advocate the use of 'Centor' or 'FeverPAIN' scores to direct treatment in primary care but these are less useful for the more severe cases typically presenting to an otolaryngologist. Infectious mononucleosis necessitates a blood film, liver function tests and serology testing (or Paul–Bunnell test). There is no role for antiviral medication but steroids may help reduce inflammation if airway compromise is threatened.

> The abdomen should be palpated for hepatosplenomegaly and the patient advised to avoid contact sports for 6 weeks if present.

GABHS is best treated with penicillin for 10 days. Clarithromycin and erythromycin are second-line agents. Treatment of asymptomatic carriers of GABHS is needed in a few select situations. Amoxicillin must be avoided as this will cause a salmon-coloured maculopapular rash in a patient infected with EBV.

What are the complications of tonsillitis?

Localised suppurative complications include peritonsillar, parapharyngeal and retropharyngeal abscesses.

Systemic non-suppurative complications include scarlet fever, rheumatic fever and post-streptococcal glomerulonephritis.

What are the indications for tonsillectomy?

The **Paradise criteria** for tonsillectomy are:

- Seven documented episodes in the preceding 12 months
- Five documented episodes per year for 2 consecutive years
- Three documented episodes per year for 3 consecutive years

Remember that recurrent tonsillitis is only one indication for tonsil removal. Adenotonsillar surgery is most commonly performed for OSA and the tonsil may also be excised for histological examination if there is suspicion of malignancy.

Local CCG guidelines may impose additional constraints on your practice but discussion of this may be best avoided during the FRCS examination unless that is the primary focus of the question.

What are the complications of tonsillectomy?

The most important complication is bleeding which may be intra-operative, primary (within 6–8 hours) or secondary (typically post-operative day 5–10). It is crucial to exclude a family history of clotting disorder and any abnormal bleeding or bruising in the child pre-operatively must be investigated to minimise and mitigate the risks.

Other complications include post-operative pain, infection of the tonsillar fossae, dental/oral injury, TMJ dislocation, velopharyngeal insufficiency, lingual nerve palsy and hypernasality.

Various surgical techniques can be used to remove the tonsils and you should be able to justify the technique you employ with reference to why your choice minimises the risk of complications.

You have been called to A&E to review a 5-year-old child with a large-volume oropharyngeal haemorrhage 6 days after tonsillectomy. How do you proceed?

'This is a medical emergency and simultaneous assessment and resuscitation are required following APLS guidelines. The child needs to be cared for in the resus department and I would ensure that a senior paediatrician, emergency doctor and paediatric nursing staff were involved.

After ensuring the child has a patent airway I would check his oxygen saturations, respiratory rate, pulse and blood pressure. He requires IV or intraosseous venous access for fluid resuscitation and blood products. Samples need to be drawn for urgent FBC, cross match and clotting profile.

I will inform the on-call paediatric anaesthetist and theatre team that we may need to bring this child to theatre immediately and inform the child's parents of this.

Ideally the child needs to be sitting up and leaning forwards to reduce ingestion and aspiration of blood and I would examine the oral cavity with the aid of suction. If the child is compliant I may attempt to apply pressure to the tonsillar fossa with an adrenaline-soaked swab but it is highly likely that the child will need to be intubated to protect the airway and prepare for theatre. Once intubated, a throat pack or swab can be applied and the child taken to theatre for cautery or ligation of the bleeding vessel. The child may benefit from a period of observation and optimisation on the paediatric intensive care unit post-operatively. I would aim to keep the parents informed at all stages and would submit the case to our departmental morbidity meeting'.

Paediatric haemorrhage calculations	e.g. 5-year-old
Weight (kg) = (Age + 4) × 2	(5 + 4) × 2 = 18 kg
Circulating blood volume = 80 mL/kg	80 × 18 = 1,440 mL
Fluid bolus = 20 mL/kg	20 × 18 = 360 mL
RBC unit = 10 mL/kg	10 × 18 = 180 mL

Vascular Malformations

MATTHEW ELLIS

An 8-year-old girl attends outpatient clinic with a 4-month history of right-sided neck swelling associated with a constant dull ache which has not responded to repeated courses of systemic antibiotics. In the last 2 months a blotchy purple discolouration has developed in the overlying skin.

How are vascular anomalies categorised?

The 2018 revision of the International Society for the Study of Vascular Anomalies (ISSVA) divides vascular anomalies into vascular tumours and vascular malformations. Vascular tumours may be benign, locally aggressive or malignant. Vascular malformations are a heterogeneous group with congenital abnormalities involving capillaries, arteries, veins, and lymphatics either solely or in combination. Lesions may be single or multiple and may be associated with a recognised syndrome.

Vascular anomalies				
	Vascular malformations			
Vascular tumours	Simple	Combined	Of major named vessels	Associated with other anomalies

Benign
Locally
  aggressive or
  borderline
Malignant
	Malformations:
	Capillary
	Lymphatic
	Venous
	Arteriovenous
	Primary
	  lymphedema
	Arteriovenous
	  fistula
		Capillary-venous
		Capillary lymphatic
		Capillary-arteriovenous
		Lymphatic-venous
		Capillary-lymphatic-
		  venous
		Capillary-lymphatic-
		  arteriovenous
		Capillary-venous-
		  arteriovenous
		Capillary-lymphatic-
		  venous-arteriovenous
			Affecting:
			Lymphatics
			Arteries
			Veins
			Anomalies of origin
			Course
			Number
			Length
			Diameter
			Valves
			Communication
			  (AVF)
			Persistence of
			  embryonal vessel
				Klippel–
				  Trenaunay
				  syndrome
				Parkes Weber
				  syndrome
				Servelle–
				  Martorell
				  syndrome
				Sturge–Weber
				  syndrome
				Maffucci
				  syndrome

 This table is a summary adapted from the ISSVA (2018) classification of vascular anomalies. The classification also lists provisionally unclassified anomalies and causal genes associated with each syndrome. Further reading is recommended at www.issva.org.

Important elements in the history and examination

- Family history
- Age of onset
- Progression
- Location
- Size and number of lesions
- Colour
- Palpable pulse or thrill
- Proximity to eye
- Stridor or sleep-disordered breathing
- Soft tissue hypertrophy

Lesions on the face, particularly in the ophthalmic (V1) distribution are associated with increased risk of intracranial lesions. Lesions in the mandibular (V3) and anterior neck distribution are associated with increased risk of lesions within the airway, most commonly subglottic haemangioma. About 50% of infants with such airway lesion also have a concurrent skin lesion. A child with multiple cutaneous lesions is at increased risk of further visceral lesions, particularly in the liver and gastrointestinal tract.

How would you investigate a cutaneous vascular malformation?

- FBC
- Ultrasound
- MRI for lesions which are large or in the upper half of the face
- Microlaryngoscopy if airway symptoms or lesions in the lower half of the face or anterior neck
- Echocardiography if heart murmur or signs of high-output cardiac failure

Ultrasonography with Doppler signal can provide information on the flow rate.

What are the phases of infantile haemangioma?

Presents after birth within the first year of life, initially as flat erythematous patch which rapidly proliferates over the first few months to a red nodular lesion. It continues growing for around a year before entering a static phase and slowly involuting over 2 to 3 years. Small lesions do not leave any long-term cosmetic defects.

Treatment of infantile haemangioma

 • Conservative management
• Propranolol
• Corticosteroids
• Pulsed-dye laser
• Interferon alpha and vincristine
• Surgical excision

What are the indications for intervention?

Symptoms such as pain, bleeding, thrombosis or ulceration. Mass effect to nearby structures, particularly when in proximity to the eye. High-output cardiac failure.

Conservative management is appropriate for most lesions, but it is important to be able to give a rationale for the indications for intervention.

What are the main complications of treatment with propranolol?

 • Bradycardia
• Hypotension
• Hypoglycaemic seizures
• Bronchospasm

Propranolol treatment is usually started at a low dose which is subsequently increased to reduce the risk of these complications. It is worth volunteering this and that you would involve a paediatrician.

What are the management options for lymphatic malformations?

• Observation
• Reduction of lesion size with injection sclerotherapy
• Surgery to completely or partly excise the lesion

Although venous malformations and lymphatic malformations are distinct entities, there is considerable overlap in their treatment. They do not resolve spontaneously.

Which syndromes are associated with vascular malformations?

 • PHACE syndrome (posterior fossa malformation, haemangioma, arterial anomalies, cardiac defects, eye abnormalities, sternal malformations)
- Hereditary haemorrhagic telangiectasia
- Klippel–Trenaunay syndrome
- Choanal atresia-lymphoedema syndrome
- PIK3CA-related overgrowth syndrome
- Blue rubber bleb nevus syndrome
- Sturge–Weber syndrome

COMMON RHINOLOGY AND FACIAL PLASTICS VIVA TOPICS

EDITED BY HESHAM SALEH

8

- Acute sinonasal infections
- Allergic rhinitis and nasal steroids
- Anosmia
- Chronic rhinosinusitis
- CSF rhinorrhoea
- Endoscopic sinus surgery
- Epistaxis
- Facial flaps and reconstruction
- Facial pain
- Fungal sinusitis
- Hereditary haemorrhagic telangiectasia
- Keloids
- Olfactory neuroblastoma
- Pinnaplasty
- Septal perforation
- Septorhinoplasty
- Sinonasal tumours
- Skin cancer

Acute Sinonasal Infections

MOHIEMEN ANWAR

Please describe this image

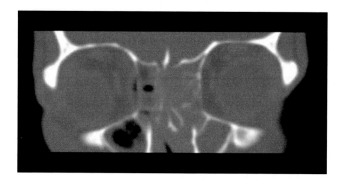

'This is a CT scan in a coronal plane across the orbit and paranasal sinuses with evidence of pansinusitis. On the right there is evidence of a gas-filled cavity in the medial-orbital wall across the lamina papyracea with an elevated and thickened periosteum displacing the globe inferolaterally, raising suspicion of peri-orbital cellulitis and subperiosteal abscess.

This is a surgical emergency and should be dealt with urgently; otherwise there is a significant risk to vision. The air bubbles and the air/fluid level on the right maxillary sinus and right ethmoid sinus are highly suggestive of an acute sinus infection with gas-forming bacteria. This scan is a non-contrast scan, ideally if suspecting an abscess formation, a contrast CT of the sinuses and orbit is preferred'.

Ensure early on that the examiners are aware that you recognise this to be a surgical emergency with urgent action needed.

What is the orbital septum?

The orbital septum is a fibrous layer of tissue that separates the skin from the globe and acts as a barrier to infection. It is formed by:

- Superiorly: From the periosteum of the orbital rim and in continuation with the levator palpebrae superioris aponeurosis
- Inferiorly: Lower part of the tarsal plate

Who should be involved in the management of this patient?

This is a surgical emergency with a risk of losing vision. Management needs an MDT approach including:

- ENT
- Ophthalmology
- Anaesthetics
- Paediatrics (if appropriate)
- Radiology
- Infectious diseases

Important elements in the history

- URTI, sinusitis, previous sinusitis, recent or current antibiotics
- Headache, facial pain, unilateral versus bilateral symptoms
- Duration of swelling and symptoms, deterioration, response to treatment
- General health and fitness for surgery
- Allergies, medications and timing of last meal

Examination

- Examine the eye urgently. With ophthalmology, assess colour vision, acuity, movement, proptosis, ophthalmoplegia, and fundoscopy to assess the optic disc.

- This is an ophthalmic emergency treated by ENT surgeons in **conjunction** with ophthalmology. Be prepared to talk about testing colour vision and acuity with Ishihara and Snellen charts, respectively. Nowadays, apps exist on mobile phones for both – show examiners that you are aware of them. According to Kollner's rule, disease affecting the optic nerve tends to cause red-green colour defects (i.e. red desaturation).

- Examine the nose for mucopurulent pus and polyps.
- Neurological examination in view of the risk of cavernous sinus thrombosis.
- Afferent papillary eye reflexes for CNIII.

Investigations

- Bloods, IV access, CRP, WCC, ESR
- CT with contrast is the usual first line imaging modality
- MRI if CN palsies and cavernous sinus thrombosis suspected or CNS involvement

When would you arrange a scan?
- If there are any eye signs beyond mild redness and swelling of the periorbita (preseptal cellulitis), i.e. proptosis, ophthalmoplegia, pain on eye movement, impaired acuity, or colour vision.

- Undetermined vision status e.g. inability to open the eye or perform an assessment.
- Lack of any clinical improvement following 36–48 hours of appropriate IV antibiotics.
- Infection in the only seeing eye.

Surgical intervention is required when a collection is identified

- Open approach: This is the gold standard in children. Use a modified Lynch Howarth brow line incision with a notch (seagull incision), down to periosteum, find the lacrimal crest, dissect the subperiosteal plane with a Freer elevator until the abscess cavity is found, washout, and leave a corrugated drain.

Remember the rule of 24 mm, 12 mm, 6 mm from the lacrimal crest, anterior ethmoid artery, posterior ethmoid artery, and optic nerve, respectively.

- Endoscopic approach: In adults, this approach might be considered though there is risk of bleeding and oedema making surgery more technically challenging. The aim is to open the ethmoid sinuses up to the lamina papyracea and drain the abscess and also conduct maxillary sinus washout. The patient should be closely monitored post-operatively. If there is failure to clinically improve then revision open approach surgery is recommended.

A joint surgical procedure with ophthalmology/neurosurgery may be considered depending on the location of the collection.

What is stage 5 in Chandler's classification and how would you manage it?

Cavernous sinus thrombosis: This is an emergency that should be managed promptly in either an intensive care unit or neuro-HDU setting. MDT approach is essential in management (neurosurgery, ophthalmology, otolaryngology, anaesthetic, intensive care, microbiology, radiology).

- 70% is caused by *Staphylococcus aureus. Streptococcus* is the second commonest organism. Other pathogens include Gram negative and rare fungal infections. An IV antibiotic that crosses the blood–brain barrier is needed e.g. ceftazidime or ceftriaxone for 3–4 weeks.
- Consider anti-coagulation, but this is an area of controversy.

 A Cochrane review (Countinho 2011) found two small trials with limited benefit over placebo, but generally low risk of complications

- Very rarely orbital decompression is needed to reduce severely elevated intraocular pressure. Surgery may also be needed to obtain microbiology samples if blood cultures fail to identify organisms
- Very rarely bilateral tying off the internal jugular veins is undertaken to reduce the risk of infected thrombus emboli to lung and peripheral vessels
- Complications
  - Elevated intraocular pressure and central vein thrombosis leading to optic nerve ischaemia and blindness
  - Intracranial infections

- Septic emboli
- The mortality rate has been quoted at 50%

What is Pott's puffy tumour and how do you manage it?

'Pott's puffy tumour is forehead swelling secondary to a frontal sinus subperiosteal abscess formation caused by frontal sinusitis and dehiscence of the anterior table of the frontal sinus'.

Management consists of:

- Prolonged broad spectrum IV antibiotics with a good blood–brain barrier penetration e.g. ceftriaxone for 6 weeks
- Nasal decongestants and nasal douching
- Regular neuro observation, watching for signs of meningitis
- MDT approach management (neurosurgery, otolaryngology, microbiology)
- Surgery is always indicated:
  - Endoscopic frontal sinus surgery
    - Draf procedure
      I. Uncinectomy and removal of the agger nasi cells to clear frontal recess

A Draf 1 procedure will usually be sufficient.

      IIa. Opening of frontal sinus from lamina to middle turbinate
      IIb. Opening the frontal sinus from lamina to septum (requires drilling)
      III. Modified Lothrop (drilling out the frontal sinuses removing from the central bony septum) (lamina to lamina across the septum and posteriorly to first olfactory fibres and anteriorly to anterior table)
    - Balloon sinuplasty may be considered in appropriate cases
  - Open approach

This is only indicated if there is an extra-dural abscess.

    - Frown-line incision for direct drainage of abscess
    - Frontal sinus trephine
    - Frontal sinus obliteration
    - Joint procedure with neurosurgery via a bicoronal approach including osteoplastic flap, removal of posterior table, and total cranialisation of frontal lobe and sealing off the drainage pathway with a pericranial flap or fascia lata graft

Allergic Rhinitis and Nasal Steroids

THOMAS JACQUES

What investigation is illustrated here? How is it performed and read?

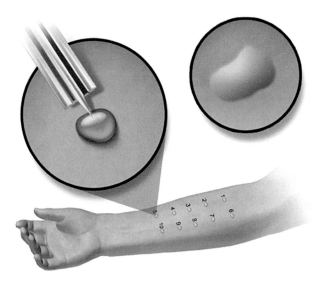

The management of rhinitis is fairly straightforward, but it is possible to get thrown by the examiners focussing on a more peripheral detail like this. Ensure that you know how tests are performed and remember to structure your answer. Give an answer that anticipates some of the possible sub-questions you may be asked.

'This is a diagram of a skin-prick allergy test, which is used to test for sensitisation to multiple allergens. A sterile lancet is used to prick the skin through a drop of allergen suspension. In addition, a positive control of histamine and a negative control of the diluent used to preserve the allergen extract are tested. Excess solution is then removed with a tissue. After 10 to 15 minutes, the results are read. A positive result is a wheal that is 3 mm or more larger than the negative control'.

Please comment on the result of this skin prick test.

DATE	MEDICAL HISTORY		SKIN PRICK TESTS		
29.11.1	Asthma: *Yes*		Risks and benefits explained		
	Hay fever or rhinitis: – *Yes* – *runny blocked nose both sides.*		Antihistamines in last 3 days? ☐ Yes ☑ No		
	Eczema *Intermittent*		Time of test: *0925* Read at: *0940.*		
	FAMILY HISTORY				
	Asthma *father, brother*		Negative control	1	—
	Hayfever or rhinitis *father brother.*				
	Eczema *Brother*		House dust mite	2	*10 mm*
	MEASURES				
	Height:	cm	Mixed tree pollens	3	*10 mm*
	Weight:	kg			
	BP:	mm Hg	Birch pollen	4	*10 mm*
	PEF:	L / min			
	NIPF:	L / min			
	☐ EXHALED NITRIC OXIDE		Mixed grass pollens	5	*5*
	Upper airway (L) (R) (500-850 ppb)		Alternaria	6	—
	Lower airway (0-20 ppb)				
	☐ RESPIRATORY FUNCTION		Aspergillus	7	—
	FEV, FER				
	FVC PEF				
	☐ NEZ DU VIN / 6		Cat epithelia	8	*8*
	☐ DIETITIAN CONSULTATION				
			Dog epithelia	9	*8*
	☑ NURSE CONSULTATION *leaflets given to patient for hayfever housedust + pet allergies*		Positive control	10	*6.*

'This patient has been noted to suffer from rhinitis and asthma, with a family history of both. In this case, the patient is sensitised to multiple allergens, including house dust mite, tree, birch and grass pollens, and cat and dog. The negative control shows no reaction and the positive control shows a 6 mm wheal'.

Note the use of 'sensitised' not 'allergic', which is a clinical diagnosis.

What would you need to ensure about the patient before they can be sent for this test?

- ☑ Ensure that the patient is not on any medications that interfere with the result: antihistamines (stop for 72 hours), topical steroid creams, tricyclics.
- Exercise caution in: unstable asthma, beta-blockers or ACE inhibitors, pregnant patients, history of anaphylaxis.
- Resuscitation facilities and appropriately trained staff must be available.
- Consider conditions that interfere with the result: Dermatographia.

What would you do if the patient was unable to have a skinprick test?

'If the patient was unable to have a skinprick allergy test, or if the results were equivocal, I would request a blood test for serum specific IgE for common aeroallergens'.

How would you manage this patient?

Remember that all you have been given is an investigation result. Rhinitis is a clinical syndrome which has many potential allergic, inflammatory and non-inflammatory causes. It is important to use a structured answer format, for example:

'This patient may have allergic rhinitis. I would start by taking a history of their allergic and nasal symptoms; specifically nasal blockage, rhinorrhoea, sneezing, itching and ocular symptoms. I would ask whether their symptoms are seasonal or provoked by exposure to other allergens such as dust or pets. I would ask whether they had a history of asthma and about their current asthma control. I would take a full past medical and drug history, ask about any family history of atopy or allergy, and their smoking and occupational history'.

After undertaking history and examination (remember external stigmata of allergy, including nasendoscopy), request appropriate investigations – **skinprick tests**, and in some cases consider FBC, immunoglobulins, ANCA and ESR.

Management typically consists of:

- Allergen avoidance (read about house dust mite precautions)
- Saline nasal douching (all patients)
- Second-generation antihistamine (particularly in mild intermittent AR; good for sneezing/itching)
- Intranasal steroid spray (long-term in perennial mod-severe AR; good for all symptoms)
- Combination steroid-topical antihistamine spray (second-line if poor control on steroid-only spray)

 Read the BSACI and ARIA guidelines for classification and algorithms for management of rhinitis, particularly so that you are familiar with non-allergic causes and the differences in management.

Are systemic steroids ever indicated in the treatment of allergic rhinitis?

'Only in cases of crises e.g. no response to standard treatment during school/university exams'.

Your patient says they are worried about taking their mometasone spray long term, and that the spray causes stinging and irritation. How would you advise them?

'I would reassure the patient that mometasone- and fluticasone-based sprays have very low systemic bioavailability, and that there is no evidence that they can cause systemic steroid-related side effects, even with long-term use. If they remained concerned, I would consider treatment with non-steroid medication, or reducing the dose'.

Most steroid nasal sprays contain a preservative called benzalkonium chloride, which in some patients can cause irritation. Flixonase nasules (fluticasone propionate drops) can be used as a substitute as they do not contain this constituent.

The patient has tried an antihistamine, combined fluticasone-azelastine nasal spray and saline irrigation for several months, but their symptoms are still very severe when in a dusty environment. They work in construction and cannot avoid all dust. What else could you consider?

- Compliance and technique advice
- Trial of another antihistamine (e.g. fexofenadine)
- Ipratropium bromide spray (if rhinorrhoea is the main symptom)
- Montelukast (if comorbid asthma)
- Sodium cromoglycate eye drops (for ocular symptoms)
- Optimise asthma management ('I would consider involving a colleague in respiratory medicine…')
- Immunotherapy ('I would refer the patient to a consultant allergist to consider…')

Immunotherapy is a disease-modifying treatment used in patients with proven sensitisation to tree or grass pollen or house dust mite (most commonly in the UK), with severe symptoms not responding to other treatments. Two forms are available: subcutaneous immunotherapy (SCIT) and sublingual immunotherapy (SLIT). In SCIT, the patient has to attend a medical facility for each injection because of a higher risk of anaphylaxis. Weekly injections are given during a build-up phase, followed by monthly injections for 3–5 years. In SLIT, the first dose is given under medical supervision. The patient then takes a daily sublingual tablet every day for 3 years.

Here is a handy list of intranasal medications that we commonly prescribe:

Beconase	Beclometasone	50 mcg per spray
Nasonex	Mometasone furoate	50 mcg per spray
Flixonase	Fluticasone propionate	50 mcg per spray
Flixonase nasules	Fluticasone propionate	400 mcg per nasule
Pirinase	Fluticasone propionate	50 mcg per spray
Avamys	Fluticasone furoate	27.5 mcg per spray
Rhinolast	Azelastine	140 mcg per spray
Dymista	F.P./azelastine	50/137 mcg per spray
Rhinocort	Budesonide	32 mcg per spray
Rinatec	Ipratropium bromide	21 mcg per spray
Nasacort	Triamcinolone acetonide	3.575 mg per spray

Anosmia

MARK FERGUSON

A patient presents unable to smell, what are the key features in the history?

 • Duration of disturbance in sense of smell
- Is it anosmia or hyposmia?
- Was the onset sudden or gradual? If sudden – is there a history of head injury or URTI?
- Background of rhinitis or CRS (with or without nasal polyps)
- Medications – codeine, carbimazole, methotrexate, metronidazole
- Other medical conditions – Alzheimer's, Parkinson's, MS, Kallmann syndrome, Turner syndrome, metabolic and endocrine disorders
- Is smell a crucial part of the patient's occupation or hobbies?
- Are there smoke detectors in the house?

What would you expect to find on examination?

Look for evidence of rhinitis/CRS/polyps

Quite likely nothing of note but you should offer to undertake a full rhinological examination.

What further investigations might you do?

- Consider CT sinuses if evidence of polyps or CRS or gradual onset.
- Consider MRI sinuses and brain to look for a central cause (anterior cranial fossa lesions).
- Be aware of smell tests such as UPSIT and Sniffin' Sticks.
- Blood might include U&E, LFT, TFT, autoimmune and syphilis screen, B12, folate, magnesium, calcium, zinc.

If pushed on what is the best imaging, opt for MRI sinuses and brain to exclude space-occupying lesions in the brain or superior nasal cavity.

What are potential causes of anosmia?

Often no cause is found.

The list is long but here are some to know:

 • Rhinitis
- CRS with and without polyps
- Head injury leading to brain damage
- URTI (viral)
- Tumours of anterior cranial fossa
- Normal process of ageing
- Dementia (can be an early sign)
- GPA (granulomatosis with polyangitis)
- Toxins
- Epilepsy

How would you manage this patient if no cause for anosmia is identified following investigations?

- Smell training (Professor Hubel, TU Dresden).
- Support groups e.g. Fifth Sense.
- If loss of smell is recent, you may offer guarded reassurance that there might be some improvement over time in some cases.
- Possibly (depending on availability) refer to your local anosmia clinic.
- Counsel the patient around steps that need to be taken to adapt to the hazards of anosmia. For instance, avoiding expired food and obtaining household smoke detectors.

Chronic Rhinosinusitis

MARK FERGUSON

Describe this image

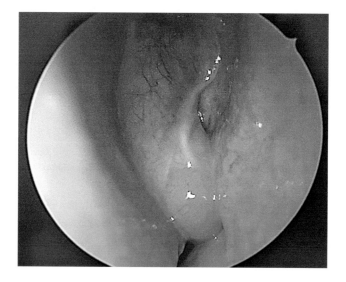

'*This is an endoscopic view of a left nasal cavity demonstrating a polyp filling the nose. This is grade 4 nasal polyposis and is consistent with CRS with nasal polyposis but I would want to examine the other side of the nasal cavity and check that this is not a solitary polyp*'.

This topic will be straightforward once you have read the latest EPOS guidelines and assimilated them into your management. For the higher marks, read the current evidence for the latest topical and surgical treatments.

How is CRS with or without polyps defined in an adult?

- Inflammation of the nose and paranasal sinuses with two or more symptoms, one of which should be nasal congestion or rhinorrhoea/post-nasal drip.
- +/− Reduced sense of smell OR facial pain
- *And either*: Endoscopic signs of nasal polyps and/or oedema of the middle meatus and/or mucopurulent discharge from the middle meatus.
- *And/or*: CT evidence of sinus disease

Symptoms should be present for more than 3 months.

What are the other pertinent features in the history and examination?

- Allergies to common aeroallergens
- Previous nasal surgery
- Current nasal medications

Past medical history:

- Asthma
- Aspirin sensitivity
- Cystic fibrosis
- Allergic fungal sinusitis
- PCD

Drug history:

- Oral steroids in the past and in the last year?
- If asthma – biologics?

Occupation: e.g. dusty environment and are there any known allergies?

Examination:

- Anterior rhinoscopy and endoscopy – polyps?
  - Meltzer clinical scoring system
    - 0 – No visible polyps
    - 1 – Confined to the middle meatus
    - 2 – Polyps occupying the middle meatus
    - 3 – Polyps extending beyond the middle meatus
    - 4 – Polyps completely obstructing the nasal cavity

How does the definition of CRS in a child differ?

Cough replaces reduced smell as a symptom.

Polyps in children are due to cystic fibrosis unless proven otherwise (e.g. the extremely rare Woakes syndrome).

How would you treat a patient like this?

 Be familiar with the EPOS 2012 guidelines. *Rhinology Supplement* 2012;23:1–298.

- Intranasal steroid and alkaline nasal douching.
- Add in an anti-histamine if allergic to aeroallergens.
- Review the patient after 6 weeks – if no improvement, consider escalation of treatment.
- E.g. stronger intranasal steroid – fluticasone propionate 400 mcg nasules.
- Or 1 week course of oral prednisolone (common practice for grade 3/4 polyps).
- And/or antibiotics
  - High IgE/polyps – doxycycline 100 mg once a day for 3 weeks
  - IgE normal/no polyps – clarithromycin 250 mg twice a day for 2 weeks
- If no improvement on maximal medical therapy, consider CT sinuses with a view to endoscopic sinus surgery.

What other treatments are available?

If the patient has asthma requiring over four admissions to hospital in a year then may be a candidate for biologics (humanised monoclonal antibody anti-IgE or anti IL-5).

What are the benefits of surgery?

- Reduce nasal obstruction
- Facilitate intranasal steroid use
- May improve nasal discharge
- Manage expectations around any improvement of smell

What risks would you consent to for a patient undergoing endoscopic sinus surgery?

Bleeding, infection, pain, CSF leak (less than 1%), orbital trauma (less than 1%), recurrence, need for further surgery, permanent anosmia (less than 1%).

CSF Rhinorrhoea

MOHIEMEN ANWAR

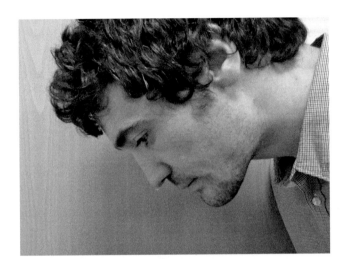

Can you describe what you can see in the above image?

'This is a picture of a patient leaning forward with evidence of clear nasal discharge. My differential diagnosis would include CSF rhinorrhoea; however, I would like to exclude more common causes of nasal discharge like rhinitis and rhinosinusitis'.

> If the patient was overweight, and after excluding all other causes of rhinorrhoea including CSF rhinorrhoea secondary to trauma, skull base fractures and surgery, one should consider and investigate the possibility of benign intracranial hypertension (BIH).

'For a definitive diagnosis of CSF leak, I would ask the patient to collect the discharge in a pre-labelled sterile pot and would send the fluid to the lab to be tested for beta-2 transferrin/tau protein; some labs would also perform beta-trace protein'.

What important points in the history and examination would help in your differential diagnosis?

- History

- Surgery including neurosurgical and otology, trauma, sinonasal symptoms, duration, rule out – rhinitis: vasomotor, gustatory rhinorrhoea etc.
- History of straining, coughing, constipation, prostatic hypertrophy
- Complications: history of headache, fever, neck rigidity, lethargy, CN palsy

- Examination

- Obese, female (BIH)
- Ear examination, CN examination and full rhinological examination including rigid nasal endoscopy. It may be possible to delineate the anatomical site of the CSF leak
- Examine for complications including CN paralysis and CNS signs (meningism, cerebral sinus thrombosis)

How would you manage this patient if the result confirms CSF rhinorrhoea?

Following history and examination and initial basic investigations including blood (FBC, WBC, CRP):

- Bed rest at 45-degree head elevation
- Stool softeners/laxatives
- Neurosurgical review
- Imaging (see later)

Assuming this patient had no history of trauma or surgery what imaging would you order for this patient, if any?

'To identify the site of the leak, I would like to start by ordering high definition CT sinuses and skull base, looking for any bony defects or evidence of air/fluid levels within the sinuses. I would also like to order MRI scan at the same time to assess for an encephalocele, intracranial pathology and hydrocephalus. MRI would help in the diagnosis of BIH'.

Intraoperative intrathecal fluorescein is indicated if CT and MRI do not show the defect or multiple defects are suspected.

What are the MRI signs of BIH?

- Patulous optic nerve due to dilated subarachnoid space around the nerve
- Flattening of the globe posteriorly
- Empty sella/slit-like ventricles turcica
- Prominent and enlarged Meckel's cave

What is the treatment of CSF rhinorrhoea?

There are few common areas to discuss here, first: the question of prophylactic antibiotics to prevent meningitis – make a decision and be able to justify it. There is no strong evidence to support prophylactic antibiotic use.

Another decision is whether to insert a lumbar drain or not. This is also very controversial and not indicated in primary cases, except possibly for proven high-pressure BIH. Be able to discuss the pros and cons and the significance of having neurosurgical cover and post-procedure care available. Always be sure to state that the management of CSF leak is in an MDT setting.

Conservative

Conservative management (45-degree bed rest and stool softeners to avoid straining) is only indicated before definitive repair or if there are contraindications for surgical management. Leaks will often close by healing of sinus mucosa, however the dura does not spontaneously repair. An approximate overall 19% risk of meningitis therefore mandates surgical repair.

- Surgical:
  - MDT approach with neurosurgical colleagues
  - Endoscopic versus open (endoscopic is the accepted method of repair in the majority of cases)
    - Depends on size, site, cause and resources (e.g. an experienced endoscopic sinus/ skull base surgeon)
  - Three-layer technique
    - Autologous dural cover (temporalis fascia, fascia lata) versus synthetic (duraGen, permacol)
    - Septal cartilage
    - For small defects, DuraSeal/Tisseel can be used and the nasal cavity packed with Nasopore. Cuffed catheters are reserved for large defects after skull base surgery.
    - For larger defects, posterior-septal nasal flap repair (Hadad flap) based on nasoseptal artery (branch of SPA)

Endoscopic Sinus Surgery

MOHIEMEN ANWAR

Please describe this image

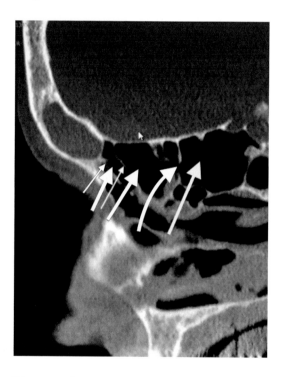

'*This is a non-contrast CT scan in the sagittal plane through the level of the sinonasal cavity and anterior skull base. The most obvious abnormality is evidence of frontal sinus opacification. I would need the axial or coronal sections to establish laterality and the status of the other sinuses*'.

At this point, you may either continue to identify each marked sinus or wait for the examiners to ask specifically.

- First arrow: Uncinate process (first lamella)
- Second arrow: Ethmoid bulla (second lamella)
- Third arrow: The vertical insertion of the middle turbinate
- Fourth arrow: Anterior ethmoid
- Fifth arrow: Basal lamella (third lamella)
- Sixth arrow: Posterior ethmoid

What are the other two sinonasal lamellae?

- Superior turbinate (fourth lamella)
- Supreme turbinate (fifth lamella) – this is extremely rare

It is important to have a system to describe the findings of a CT scan of the paranasal sinuses.

CLOSET is one commonly used system:

C: Cribriform plate and carotid artery

L: Lamina

O: Optic nerve and Onodi cell (sphenoethmoidal) (not shown here and best seen on the axial plane)

S: Sphenoid

E: Ethmoids and ethmoid artery (Kennedy's nipple)

T: Teeth and maxillary sinuses

The coronal plane is used to assess:

- Septum
- Optic nerve and proximity to lamina
- Intracranial pathology
- Onodi cells, which appear as a transverse septation of the sphenoid sinuses

The sagittal plane is best for assessing:

- The shape of the frontal sinuses: the bony peaks, anterior and posterior tables and fronto-ethmoidal cells
- Skull base level and orientation
- Onodi cells (also seen on the axial views)

What is the agger nasi cell and what is its significance?

An agger nasi cell is the most anterior ethmoid air cell, lying anterolateral to the frontal recess and anterior to the vertical insertion of the middle turbinate. It is present in almost 90% of adult sinuses. It is an anatomical landmark for the frontal recess.

Other clinically significant sinus variants include:

- Haller cell: Infraorbital ethmoid air cell. Present in 20% of adult sinuses.
- Onodi cell: Sphenoethmoidal cell. The most posterior ethmoid cell that extends posterolateral to the sphenoid. It is significant for its proximity to the optic nerve and ICA.

Is the agger nasi cell part of the fronto-ethmoidal cells?

No. Fronto-ethmoidal cells, also known as Kuhn cells, are anterior ethmoid cells that have migrated towards the frontal sinus. There are four types:

I.   Single cell superior to agger nasi cell

II. Multiple cells superior to agger nasi cell

III. Giant single cell extending into the frontal sinus

IV. An isolated cell confined to the frontal sinus

On the axial scan image, can you grade the level of the skull base?

According to Keros classification it is grade III

- Keros I. 1–3 mm
- Keros II. 4–7 mm
- Keros III. 8–16 mm
- Keros IV. Asymmetrical

In the same image, if we assume that both the frontal and the sphenoid sinuses are completely opacified, can you score these CT findings?

According to Lund-McKay index score, I would score this as 23/24.

0: No disease

1: Partial disease

2: Complete opacification

Maxillary, frontal, ant. ethmoid, post. ethmoid, sphenoid to be scored 0, 1, or 2.

Osteomeatal complexes to be scored 0 if open and 2 if blocked (no 1 score).

Based on that and the information provided, only the left maxillary sinus can be scored as 1, the rest all 2, to a total score of 23/24.

What is the SNOT-22 and what are the minimal and maximum scores?

In this situation, you may either quote your own figures, though hopefully your rate of rare complications will be nil.

Sino Nasal Outcome Test Questionnaire. Scores 0 (no problem) to 5 (problem as bad as it can be) for 22 questions related to the nose e.g. sense of smell, nasal obstruction. The minimum score is 0 and the maximum is 110.

 Refer to the literature for examples of application of the questionnaire:

Philpott et al. *BMJ Open.* 2015;5(4):e006680

Hopkins et al. *Clin Otolaryngol.* 2006 Oct;31(5):390–8.

When consenting patients for FESS, what complication rates do you quote?

- Bleeding rate 5%
- CSF leak rate 2:3000
- Eye complications 7:3000

It may be necessary to describe your own surgical experience of endoscopic sinus surgery for example indications, technical approaches and theatre setup (position, draping, instruments, techniques etc.)

What is Moffett's solution?

- 1 mL of 1/1000 adrenaline
- 1 mL of 10% cocaine
- 2 mL of 8.4% sodium bicarbonate

Epistaxis

SAMIT UNADKAT

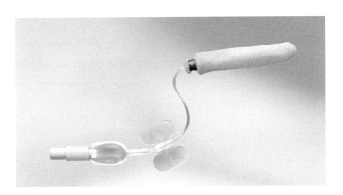

Where have you seen this being used?

'This is a Rapid Rhino nasal pack used in the management of epistaxis. The pack is dipped in water for around 30 seconds and inserted along the nasal floor. The cuff is inflated with air to help tamponade the bleeding'.

> Often examiners will start with an entry level question such as this before getting to the meat of the topic. Do not be phased, answer succinctly, and wait for the next question.

An elderly patient presents to the emergency department with recurrent epistaxis and is reviewed by your senior house officer. They have been discharged 2 days previously with a similar epistaxis. He would like something definitive. How would you manage this scenario?

> This is a typical scenario that you would encounter at work. The examiner here is looking for a stepwise and systematic approach.

In the Emergency department, the patient is likely to be more unstable than if they presented to clinic with recurrent epistaxis and your management would differ.

- ABC measures
- Oxygen saturation monitoring
- Wide bore IV access
- FBC, U+E
- Group & save and clotting screen
- Direct pressure and an oral/topical ice pack
- Wear protective equipment
- Obtain suction, a headlight and assistance

Only once adequate control has been made should you move on to taking a full history:

- Duration of epistaxis
- Frequency
- Site (bilateral/unilateral)
- Previous interventions
- Any loss of consciousness
- Trauma
- Recent surgery
- History of hypertension/IHD/coagulopathies/malignancy
- Bruising, anticoagulation/antiplatelet therapy
- Family history (think HHT, vWD, haemophilia).

If the patient is unstable and bleeding despite conservative measures, consider the following in a stepwise approach:

- Cautery with $AgNO_3$ +/− Naseptin and Nasopore (or similar dissolvable packing)
- Anterior nasal packing with Merocel or Rapid Rhino
- FloSeal
- BIPP
- Foley catheter + BIPP

Invariably, whatever can go wrong, will go wrong in the scenario given in the exam, so be prepared to escalate your treatment beyond the aforementioned. Aside from the surgical aspect, think about the patient's general health and involving the medical team, haematologists, obtaining an ECG, finding out when the patient last ate and drank and an anaesthetic review. Consider an HDU bed as elderly patients often have numerous comorbidities. There is reasonable evidence that tranexamic acid decreases the number of rebleeding events. It is likely that the patient will need a rapid sequence intubation so be able to describe it.

If all conservative measures have failed, how would you arrest the bleeding?

'After appropriate resuscitation and obtaining informed consent, I would perform a bilateral endoscopic SPA ligation. After decongesting the nose, I would infiltrate using a spinal needle and perform an uncinectomy and middle meatal antrostomy to visualise the posterior wall of the maxillary antrum. I would raise a mucoperiosteal flap until the crista ethmoidalis was encountered. The SPA is immediately posterior to this. Sometimes the crista needs to be curetted. I would use endoscopic bipolar diathermy to cauterise the branches and continue until I reach the face of the sphenoid'.

Radiological embolisation is an alternative to surgery in cases of intractable epistaxis.

Why do you perform a *bilateral* SPA ligation?

There is 15% cross-over of the blood supply.

If the patient had suffered a traumatic epistaxis, would your management differ?

This is an area of controversy as traditional teaching suggests that the anterior ethmoidal artery is the first artery that ought to be ligated. However, many rhinologists will still carry out an endoscopic SPA ligation first, even in trauma cases. The patient may also need a manipulation under anaesthetic nose so don't forget to discuss that.

 Be able to describe the external approach to ligating the anterior ethmoid artery and IMAX

Remember the anterior lacrimal crest is 24 mm to the anterior ethmoid artery which is 12 mm to the posterior ethmoidal artery which is 6 mm to the optic nerve.

Facial Flaps and Reconstruction

THOMAS JACQUES

This patient presents to your clinic with a lesion on the tip of his nose. What is the best surgical treatment for this lesion?

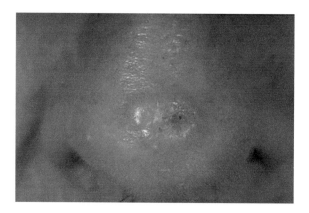

'This is a clinical photograph of a patient's nasal tip. There is a lesion occupying a large proportion of the nasal tip subunit which is consistent with a BCC. Assuming the patient was fit for surgical management, I would recommend excision with a 5 mm margin, as the nose is a high-risk area'.

Management of BCC – Options:

- Conservative
- Non-surgical
    - Cryotherapy
    - Curettage
    - Photodynamic therapy
    - Radiotherapy
    - 5% Imiquimod
- Surgical
    - Wide local excision
    - Mohs micrographic surgery

What are the reconstructive options for this patient?

'It may improve the eventual cosmesis to enlarge the defect to include the remainder of the tip subunit. Anticipating the size and position of the defect, I would select the most appropriate option from the reconstructive ladder. Secondary intention healing is possible but undesirable *because of the poor cosmesis and prolonged healing process. Primary closure would be impossible with this size of defect on the nose. A full thickness skin graft would be obvious and unlikely to give a good colour or texture match but could be acceptable if the patient was unfit for more prolonged surgery. Considering local random pattern flaps, the defect would be too large for a bilobed flap or nasolabial flap. The optimal reconstructive option would probably be a paramedian forehead flap'.*

Describe and draw a paramedian forehead flap

- A local, axial-pattern interpolated rotation flap based on the supratrochlear vessels, ideal for large nasal defects.
- Requires at least two stages – excision and flap inset, then pedicle division 2–3 weeks later.
- Landmarks for supratrochlear vascular bundle:
  1. Above medial canthus (+/− 3 mm)
  2. 2 cm lateral to midline (+/− 3 mm)
  3. 1 cm medial to supraorbital notch
- Flap is raised approximately 1.5 cm wide, ensuring it is long enough to rotate into the defect.
- Initially elevated in the subgaleal plane. Deepened to the subperiosteal plane from 3 cm above brow.

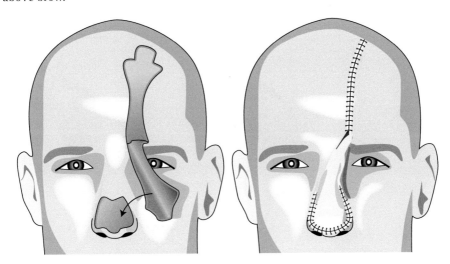

What are the layers that are affected in a full-thickness defect of the alar margin? How would you reconstruct this?

- Skin
- SMAS
- Fibro-fatty tissue and lateral crus of alar cartilage (depending on position)
- Vestibular skin/mucosa

'The skin and mucosal layers are best reconstructed with local rotational flaps. A nasolabial flap is a good option for the external flap, and mucosa can be rotated from the septum or inferior

turbinate. The reconstruction has to be supported by cartilage which reaches all the way to the alar rim to prevent notching, regardless of whether cartilage was resected. I would harvest this from the conchal bowl'.

What are the stages a skin graft goes through as it 'takes'?

1. *Fibrin adhesion*
2. *Plasmatic imbibition* (the graft survives the 24–48 hours pre-vascular stage by 'drinking' from the plasma)
3. *Revascularisation* (36 hours onwards – capillary ingrowth from bed – graft vessels anastomose to bed vessels [inosculation] – graft becomes pink)
4. *Remodelling* (4 days – restoration of normal histological architecture, replacement of fibrin glue with permanent fibrous attachment)

Important local flaps to know:

Make sure that you are familiar with the following local flaps, which you could be asked to describe and/or draw.

Nasolabial flap: Skin from the medial cheek is rotated into a defect on the nasal alar or sidewall region. The flap can be superiorly or inferiorly based. A triangle is cut at the apex to allow the defect to close in line with the nasolabial crease.

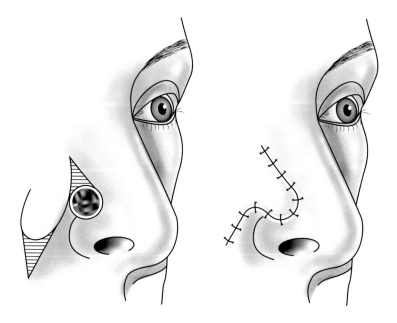

Rhomboid flap: Originally known as the Limberg flap. The defect is shaped into a rhombus. There are **four possible flaps** in each case, extending from the wider 120-degree angle of the rhombus. Choose the flap that takes the best advantage of the laxity of adjacent skin and does not impinge on vital structures.

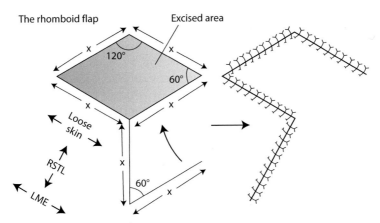

The rhomboid flap   Excised area

120°

60°

Loose
skin

RSTL

60°

LME

RSTL - relaxed skin tension line
LME - lines of maximal extensibility

Z-plasty: A Z-plasty is used to re-orient, lengthen, and irregularise a scar. This may be because the scar is causing webbing/contracture, or because it is running perpendicular to skin lines/RSTLs, making it unsightly. Multiple Z-plasties can be used to lengthen and irregularise longer scars. The amount of lengthening depends on the angles used when constructing the Z-plasty:

30 degrees = 25% longer

45 degrees = 50% longer

60 degrees = 75% longer

75 degrees = 100% longer

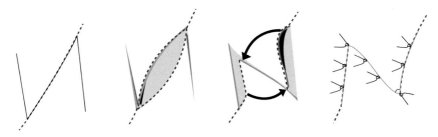

V-Y advancement: A triangle ('V') of skin is advanced as an *island* into the defect. The skin behind the advancement is closed in a line, forming the 'Y'.

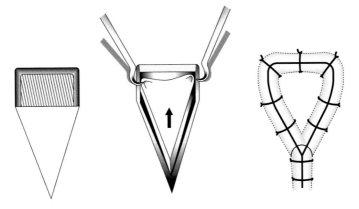

Practise drawing this flap several times as it can be challenging to get right.

Bilobed flap: A circular flap is rotated by approximately 45 degrees into the adjacent defect. A narrower ovoid flap is rotated by a further 45 degrees into the secondary defect, and the final defect is closed primarily. The centre of rotation is one radius below the defect. The total arc of rotation is 90 degrees – note that this is technically a modification of the originally described technique by Esser. The bilobed flap is often used to reconstruct small (up to 1.5 cm) defects on the lower half of the nose, or on the temporal forehead.

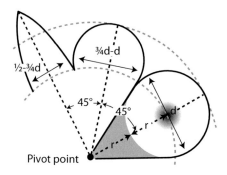

Lip flaps: Defects less than one-third of the lip width can be closed primarily in a V or W fashion. Larger defects require local tissue transfer. This may maintain orbicularis integrity, preserving function at the expense of microstomia or may transfer additional tissue into the lip region, potentially compromising function. Two examples are as follows:

- *Abbé flap*: This full-thickness flap is used to reconstruct upper or lower lip defects between one-third and two-thirds of the lip width. A wedge of the unaffected lip is rotated into the defect on its vascular attachment medially. The pedicle, which initially bridges across the mouth, is divided at 2–3 weeks. When the defect involves the oral commissure, the technique is known as the Abbé-Estlander flap. This produces rounding of the oral commissure which is revised at 2–3 weeks.

- *Karapandzic flap*: This flap is used for the reconstruction of larger midline lower or upper lip defects. It is an axial rotational flap based on superior and inferior labial arteries. It has the advantage of maintaining commissure integrity and thus oral competence, sensation, and movement, but the disadvantage of creating microstomia and relatively unsightly scarring.

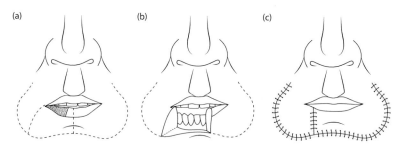

Although less likely to appear, it may also be worth familiarising yourself with the various reconstructive flaps for pinna lesions: Wedge, stellate and Antia-Buch.

Facial Pain

THOMAS JACQUES

A 45-year-old female patient presents with a year's history of facial pain. She feels an aching in her cheeks and behind her eyes. She has not responded to intranasal steroid sprays and would like more treatment for her 'sinusitis'. How would you manage this patient?

In open-ended clinical scenarios, it is important to remain systematic. However, where there is a 'key principle' that the examiners want to elicit, it can help to start with a brief statement that lets them know you understand the key issues:

'Chronic facial pain is rarely due to sinonasal disease, especially if the patient does not have the symptoms of CRS as defined by the EPOS 2012 guidelines. I would focus on eliminating sinusitis as a possible explanation for the patient's symptoms, before focussing on the cause of the patient's facial pain, which may be neurological'.

Important elements in the history

 Characteristics of facial pain: Timing, episodic or constant, debilitating or not, symmetrical or not, visual aura, lethargy/nausea/imbalance/photophobia, autonomic features, triggers.

Symptoms of rhinosinusitis: Nasal blockage, rhinorrhoea, change/decrease in sense of smell, stress, caffeine intake, analgesic use, family history of migraine.

'I would take the history concentrating on specific features of the facial pain such as...'

'I would aim to elicit any symptoms suggestive of rhinosinusitis such as ...'

'I would ask the patient about risk factors for chronic headache such as ...'

'I would then perform anterior rhinoscopy, nasendoscopy, examine the TMJ and a CN examination'.

The patient has no additional features of rhinosinusitis – what is the differential diagnosis?

You are not expected to have detailed knowledge of the management of all headache syndromes, but it is reasonable for a candidate to know about the management of common forms of headache that are confused for sinusitis (tension-type headache, midfacial segment pain, migraine).

TTH: May be *episodic* or *chronic*: Symmetrical, dull pain felt typically in frontal, bitemporal and occipital regions. Non-debilitating (cf. migraine). Treated primarily with amitriptyline (gabapentin second line).

Midfacial segment pain: Essentially similar to TTH, but the pain is felt in the retro-orbital regions, the cheeks or the nasion. This is commonly attributed to sinonasal disease. The same management as TTH.

Migraine: 4–72 hour episodes, sometimes with preceding aura. Severe, asymmetrical, throbbing pain, accompanied by systemic upset such as nausea, lethargy, photophobia or phonophobia. Most common in young women. Managed with symptomatic medication (aspirin, triptans) and prophylactic medication (pizotifen, propranolol).

TMJ pain: Aching pain around the TMJ(s), radiating to the temples or neck. May be prominent in the morning due to nocturnal bruxism. The patient may have pain on chewing or trismus.

Analgesic-overuse headache: Caused by dependence on analgesics such as paracetamol in patients with a history of TTH or migraine.

Other forms of facial pain less likely in this specific scenario:

Cluster headache: Excruciating, shorter (around 1 hour) episodes of unilateral periorbital pain, accompanied by lacrimation and a bloodshot eye. Episodes come and go in 'clusters'. Most common in young or middle-aged men.

Trigeminal neuralgia: Severe shooting pain in the distribution of V2 or V3. Carbamazepine is first-line.

Paroxysmal hemicrania: Another form of trigeminal autonomic cephalgia. Most common in women. Short-lived unilateral facial pain with autonomic features. Responds to indomethacin.

SUNCT and SUNA: Short lasting unilateral neuralgiform headache with conjunctival injection and tearing (SUNCT) and short lasting unilateral neuralgiform headache attacks with cranial autonomic symptoms (SUNA) are rare primary headache disorders that respond to subcutaneous lignocaine. Lamotrigine may be used as a preventative.

Atypical facial pain: Migratory pain, often accompanied by psychological distress. A diagnosis of exclusion.

 Read about the pharmacological management of common chronic headache/facial pain syndromes (SIGN headache guidelines, or Kamani T and Jones NS, *Clin Otolaryngol*. 2012 Jun;37[3]:207–12).

Would you request any imaging for this patient?

There is no right or wrong answer, but you must be prepared to argue your case. This is a potential answer:

'*If the patient had a typical history of a chronic headache syndrome, no red flags for malignancy and no symptoms or clinical signs of rhinosinusitis, I would not request any imaging at the first consultation. Imaging can have a role if the diagnosis is unclear, or to eliminate a sinonasal cause for the patient's pain. However, I would be mindful of the fact that there is a roughly 30% rate of incidental sinus opacification in the normal population*'.

You diagnose this lady with midfacial segment pain. How would you manage her?

- Reassure the patient.
- Explain that the pain is not due to sinus disease.
- Commence a trial of amitriptyline 10 mg nocte that can be increased up to 50 mg and ask the GP to follow-up and titrate the dose as required.
- Alternatively, seek a neurological opinion or pain clinic consultation.

Fungal Sinusitis

MOHIEMEN ANWAR

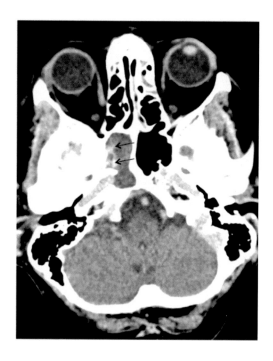

Please describe what you can see in this image

'*This is an axial contrast CT scan at the level of the orbits and sinonasal cavity. It is on soft tissue window. The arrows point to the right sphenoid sinus, demonstrating a totally opacified sinus with a double-density sign, highly suggestive of a fungal infection. The lack of bony erosions is in keeping with non-invasive fungal sinusitis, although I would examine the bone window to confirm*'.

CT sinuses should be studied systematically. Following the description of the scan and the sections, check the sinuses for opacifications, bony erosion signifying invasive fungal sinusitis, mucocele, double-density sign, orbit and any abscess formation and finally any intracranial findings of sinus thrombosis or abscess formation.

Are you aware of any classifications for sinonasal fungal infections?

Fungal infections of the sinonasal cavity can be broadly divided into invasive versus non-invasive infection, based on the infection's ability to cause bony erosion and invasion.

- Non-invasive fungal sinusitis can be further divided into two major subtypes:
  - Mycetoma 'fungal ball', typically affecting one sinus cavity, commonly the maxillary sinus and often an incidental CT finding. *Aspergillus fumigatus* is often the causative

pathogen. Patients are usually immunocompetent. It can be associated with dental infections, asthma, diabetes and granulomatous inflammatory conditions of the sinonasal cavity. CT sinuses generally reveal no bone erosion, however there may be evidence of a bony reaction (osteitis) and new bone formation due to the chronic inflammation. Typically a double-density sign may be present due to the accumulation of heavy metals in the fungal hyphae. Mycetoma produce signal voids in MRI T2-weighted scans, resembling an aerated sinus cavity. Endoscopic sinus surgery to create a wide middle meatal antrostomy will allow complete removal of the fungal ball.

○ Allergic fungal sinusitis, a disease often associated with thick mucin rich in eosinophils ('axle-grease') and positive stain for fungal infection. Patients often suffer from symptoms of CRS that are resistant to medical therapy.

The acronym 'ABCD' is a useful aide memoire for the fungi causing mycetoma – *Aspergillus fumigatus*, *Bipolaris*, *Curvularia lunata*, and *Drechslera*.

Are you aware of any diagnostic criteria for allergic fungal sinusitis?

- Bent and Kuhn criteria:
  ○ Major:
    ▪ Type-1 hypersensitivity
    ▪ Nasal polyps
    ▪ Fungal staining
    ▪ CT changes
    ▪ Eosinophilic mucin
  ○ Minor:
    ▪ Asthma
    ▪ Unilateral
    ▪ Systemic eosinophilia
    ▪ Charcot-Leyden crystals
    ▪ Fungal culture

Treatment includes initial medical therapy with systemic and topical steroids and nasal douching, if failed then FESS.

 Read the original paper by Bent and Kuhn (Bent JP, Kuhn FA. Diagnosis of allergic fungal sinusitis. *Otolaryngol Head Neck Surg* 1994;111:580–8).

- Invasive fungal sinusitis:

Acute fulminant invasive fungal sinusitis (mucormycosis).

It is important to stress to the examiners that this is a potentially fatal disease that needs to be treated aggressively.

Caused by saprophytic fungi such as *Rhizopus, Rhizomucor, Absidia and Mucor.* Immunocompromised and poorly controlled diabetic patients are at risk of this infection with a mortality rate of more than 50%. It causes an invasive infection that erodes through the bone and soft tissue of the skull base. Intracranial invasion is almost invariably fatal.

How do you investigate and manage a patient with suspected mucormycosis?

- History: Evidence of sinusitis in an unwell and immunocompromised patient is highly suspicious of mucormycosis.
- Examination: 'The black turbinate sign' on nasal endoscopy, signs of sepsis, CNS signs (e.g. reduced GCS, CN palsies)
- Radiological: Both CT and MRI are indicated for diagnosis. CT shows sinus opacification with an aggressive pattern of erosion. MRI with contrast shows sinus opacification with evidence of necrotic non-enhancing tissues, with orbital and intracranial involvement.
- Treatment: Aggressive surgical debridement with a prolonged course of systemic anti-fungals.

Which anti-fungals would you give to the patient?

Amphotericin B (1.5 mg/kg/d) or voriconazole 200 mg bd for up to 1 year.

Are there any other forms of invasive fungal sinusitis?

- Chronic invasive aspergillosis (*A. fumigatus* is the commonest. Other *Aspergillus* subtypes are *niger, flavus* and *nidulans*).
- Chronic granulomatous invasive fungal sinusitis occurs in Sudan, Egypt and Afghanistan (*Aspergillus flavus* exclusively).

Hereditary Haemorrhagic Telangiectasia

MARK FERGUSON

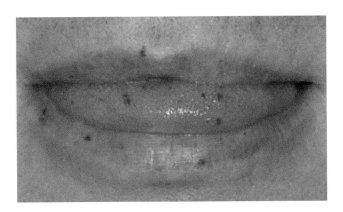

Please describe this image

'This is a clinical photograph showing telangiectasia on the lips and tongue, this is consistent with a diagnosis of hereditary haemorrhagic telangiectasia'.

In a rhinology viva, this is the diagnosis if you are presented with a photo like this or a video showing lasers being used to thermo-coagulate telangiectasia. Be concise and state the presence of the lesions and say what its most likely to be consistent with as the viva will be primarily around the management of this condition.

Do you know any diagnostic criteria?

Curaçao criteria (three or four features = definite HHT, two features = possible HHT)

1. Spontaneous recurrent epistaxis
2. Multiple telangiectasias
3. Proven visceral AVM
4. First degree family member with HHT

How do these patients present?

- Recurrent epistaxis
- GI or pulmonary bleeds
- Intracranial bleeds

Family history: Multiple first-degree relatives affected

Medications: Patients avoid anti-coagulants (if they can), nonsteroidal anti-inflammatory drugs

Examination: Multiple facial and lip telangiectasias may be present

Caution – You must be very careful when you examine the nose. Performing nasolaryngoscopy can risk triggering bleeding in the clinic setting. Examining the nose is important for clinical assessment however – use a 2.7 mm 30-degree scope which is safe as long as you don't touch the telangiectasia.

There will be telangiectasias on the anterior septum, roof of nose, and lateral wall extending back to the anterior border of the middle turbinate but no further back than that.

How are these patients managed?

Investigations can depend on the area you work but here is a suggested structure:

- Referral to HHT physician – for management of non-ENT manifestations of disease
- Bloods – FBC (baseline Hb especially if contemplating surgery)
- CT chest and abdomen looking for pulmonary and hepatic AVMs (if the patient has not had previous imaging in the last 5 years)

The head may not be scanned if there are no neurological features as management of brain AVM is typically conservative due to the risk.

Medical:

- Creams (antibiotic/emollient)
- Tranexamic acid either oral or topical as an atomised spray (for mild/moderate bleeds)
- Kaltostat placed in the nose
- Oestrogen receptor-modulating agents – tamoxifen/oestradiol creams
- Diet – salicylate low/moderate diet – temporary as no one can tolerate this for long
- Anti-VEGF inhibitors e.g. bevacizumab

Surgical:

- KTP laser (or other lasers can be used such as YAG, plasma argon) to thermo-coagulate lesions
- Septodermoplasty
- Modified Young's procedure

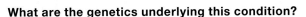

What are the genetics underlying this condition?

Five genetic subtypes are recognised. Currently it remains primarily a clinical diagnosis although there are genetic tests available for:

- *ENG* (coding for endoglin, a receptor of TGF-β1)
- *ACVRL1* (coding for Alk-1, another TGF-β1 receptor)
- *MADH4*

There are over 600 different variants that have been associated with HHT; however, over 80% of cases are due to variants in *ENG* or *ACVRL1*.

Why are the blood vessels and telangiectasias so friable?

This is thought to be due to a lack of elastin/muscle in tunica media of blood vessels and therefore vessels can't contract.

Further reading:

A treatment algorithm for the management of epistaxis in hereditary hemorrhagic telangiectasia. Lund VJ, Howard DJ. *Am J Rhinol.* 1999 Jul–Aug;13(4):319–22.

The impact of septodermoplasty and KTP laser therapy in the treatment of hereditary hemorrhagic telangiectasia-related epistaxis. *Am J Rhinol.* 2008 Mar–Apr;22(2):182–7. doi: 10.2500/ajr.2008.22.3145.

Nasal closure for severe hereditary haemorrhagic telangiectasia in 100 patients. The Lund modification of the Young's procedure: a 22-year experience. *Rhinology.* 2017 Jun 1;55(2):135–41. doi: 10.4193/Rhin16.315.

Keloids

THOMAS JACQUES

A 23-year-old lady comes to your clinic with this lesion on her right pinna which has been growing for about a year. How would you manage her?

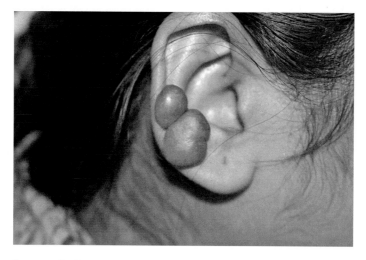

Image credit: Htirgan • CC BY-SA 3.0. https://commons.wikimedia.org/

Questions starting on a relatively specific topic will usually then be supplemented with more general questions.

'*This is a clinical photograph of a woman with a pedunculated lesion on the posterosuperior aspect of the right pinna lobule. This has the appearance of a keloid and may have occurred at the site of a previous piercing. I would take a history focussing on the onset and precipitating factors of the lesion, ask about her personal and family history of keloids, and take a full medical history. I would examine the lesion for its mobility, consistency and the size of the pedicle. It is my practice to offer intralesional surgical excision of this lesion with perioperative injection of a corticosteroid such as triamcinolone acetonide. I would warn her about the relatively high chance of recurrence*'.

Management of keloids:

(Medical treatment can be given alone or as an adjunct to surgery)

Prevention	Avoid surgery and piercings
	Treat acne aggressively
	Avoid close shaving if causing skin irritation
	Tension-free closure of wounds
Medical treatment	Steroid injection
	Compression therapy
	Silicone sheeting
	Immunomodulators: 5-fluorouracil, interferon, bleomycin
	Radiotherapy
Surgical treatment	Intralesional or extralesional excision
	Laser ablation

What is a keloid, and how does it differ from a hypertrophic scar?

Keloids are caused by a proliferation of atypical fibroblasts at the site of skin injury. This leads to excessive deposition of initially type-3 collagen, which is then replaced by type-1 collagen. The risk of keloid formation is related to skin pigmentation, with the highest risk in Afro-Caribbeans, and is most common in young adults. They are most common when a wound is not aligned with relaxed skin tension lines (RSTLs). A keloid extends beyond the margin of the original injury or scar, whereas a hypertrophic scar does not.

What are the stages of wound healing?

1. Haemostasis (occurs within minutes): fibrin deposition and platelet aggregation.
2. Inflammatory (minutes up to a week): influx of inflammatory cells which are phagocytose dead cells/pathogens.
3. Proliferative (after 2–3 days): fibroblast-mediated deposition of collagen to form granulation tissue, then re-epithelialisation.
4. Remodelling (weeks to months): gradual realignment of collagen along skin tension lines. Wound reaches 80% strength by 12 weeks.

How can you make a scar less obvious?

This is an ambiguous question: Start with basic principles of wound placement and closure, then move on to revision techniques.

- Incision design
  - Parallel to RSTLs (Ensure you can draw these on the face)
  - Camouflaged within existing skin lines (e.g. neck creases, nasolabial fold)
  - Broken lines draw the eye less readily – consider especially where crossing RSTLs

- Closure
  - Eliminate tension through undermining and multilayer closure (e.g. closing platysma carefully before skin)
  - Gentle tissue handling
  - Consider a fine (5-0 or 6-0) monofilament suture (may lessen tissue reaction)
  - Remove sutures promptly (7 days generally, 5 days maximum on face)
- Aftercare
  - Taping to lessen shearing forces
  - Sun protection
  - Moisturisation, massage
- Revision
  - Dermabrasion
  - Steroid injection
  - Pulsed-dye laser
  - Fillers/autologous fat graft (for depressed scars)
  - Elliptical scar excision and closure
  - Re-alignment: Z-plasty
  - Irregularisation: Multiple Z-plasty, W-plasty, geometric broken line repair

Olfactory Neuroblastoma

MARK FERGUSON

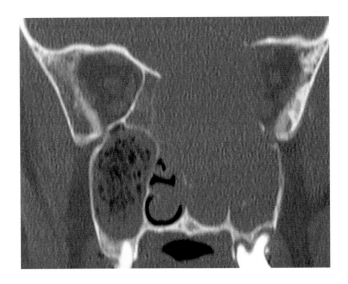

Describe this coronal CT scan

'*There is a superiorly based expansile lesion within the nasal cavity that has eroded bone and is extending into the orbit on the left. This is most consistent with a sinonasal malignancy, I'm aware there is a wide range of possible pathologies, the most common of which is SCC, but given its position within the sinonasal region this could be an olfactory neuroblastoma (also known as esthesioneuroblastoma, that arises from neuroectodermal olfactory cells) or sinonasal undifferentiated carcinoma (SNUC). I would like to arrange further imaging in the form of an MRI sinuses, and appropriate neck imaging and plan for an EUA and biopsy*'.

How do these lesions present?

 • Unilateral nasal obstruction
- Serosanguinous or blood-stained discharge
- Anosmia
- Facial pain
- Paraesthesia
- Trismus
- Epiphora
- Diplopia
- Proptosis/chemosis

What is the differential diagnosis?

 • SCC
- Adenocarcinoma
- Olfactory neuroblastoma
- Sinonasal undifferentiated carcinoma
- Neuroendocrine carcinoma
- Malignant melanoma
- ACC
- Rhabdomyosarcoma (young person)
- NK/T cell lymphoma

What investigations would you arrange?

- CT sinuses for examination of the bony anatomy
- MRI – typically shows heterogeneous intermediate signal in both T1 and T2, with variable enhancement with contrast

Imaging can be suggestive of an olfactory neuroblastoma based on location and appearance but the differential remains wide and biopsy is required.

Make sure you check the neck – up to 25% of olfactory neuroblastomas have unilateral or bilateral lymph nodes.

Is there a classification system?

- Kadish et al (1976):
  - Group A: Limited to nasal cavity
  - Group B: A + paranasal sinuses
  - Group C: Extends beyond nasal cavity and paranasal sinuses
- Chao et al. (2001) added 'Group D: Cervical nodal metastases'
- Hyam's grading is used for histological diagnosis

How would you manage this patient?

- Assuming the patient is medically fit and the tumour is surgically resectable, discuss the case in the local skull base MDT.
- Typical management involves surgical resection – endoscopic, combined (endoscopic and open), craniofacial.
- A neck dissection may be indicated.
- Post-operative radiotherapy and/or CT may be indicated.

Remember the social sequelae of the patient's anosmia. Enquire about their profession and hobbies and advise on necessary precautions.

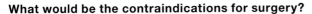

What would be the contraindications for surgery?

Absolute contraindications:

1. Invasion into cavernous sinus particularly if involving ICA
2. Massive intracranial extension

Relative contraindications:

1. Loss of both eyes
2. Loss of only seeing eye

When is endoscopic surgery inadequate for this condition?

 If orbital exenteration is needed (or through orbital periosteum)

Maxillectomy (except for medial wall)

Skin excision

Anterior and/or far lateral involvement of frontal sinus

Dura/brain involvement lateral to mid-orbital roof or lateral to optic nerve

Brain parenchyma invasion

Vascular invasion (ICA; cavernous sinus)

Optic chiasm invasion

What is the overall prognosis?

Olfactory neuroblastoma has an approximate overall 75% 5-year survival.

How are these pts followed-up?

Patients are followed-up life-long surveillance MRI and EUA+biopsy as necessary.

 Further reading:

Lund VJ, Clarke PM, Swift AC, McGarry GW, Kerawala C, Carnell D. Nose and paranasal sinus tumours: United Kingdom National Multidisciplinary Guidelines. *J Laryngol Otol.* 2016 May;130(Suppl 2):S111–8. doi: 10.1017/S0022215116000530

Lund VJ, Stammberger H, Nicolai P et al. European position paper on endoscopic management of tumours of the nose, paranasal sinuses and skull base. *Rhinol Suppl.* 2010 Jun 1;22:1–143.

Pinnaplasty

SAMIT UNADKAT

Please describe this clinical photograph

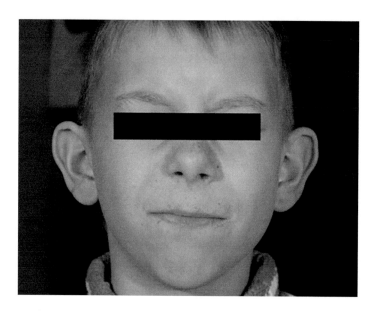

'*This is a clinical photograph, in the frontal view, of a young male demonstrating bilateral prominent ears (prominauris). There is overdevelopment of the conchal bowl and underdevelopment of the antihelical fold. Ideally I would also like to assess posterior and lateral views*'.

Note that a normal concha-mastoid angle is between 20 and 30 degrees. Prominauris is defined as an angle of greater than 40 degrees.

Be able to mark out the key anatomical landmarks of the pinna (shown below)

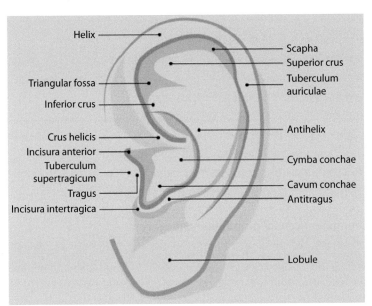

Be able to describe succinctly the embryological development of the pinna.

What are the key points to explore in the history?

- Patient and parental concerns – often the child may be oblivious at a young age
- Any history of bullying/teasing
- Impact on school performance?
- Impact on self-esteem and social anxiety?
- Comorbidities
- Congenital abnormalities

What are the options for management?

In any management of a condition question, always mention that you would start by undertaking a thorough history and examination. This scenario is yet another example that necessitates an MDT approach, including paediatric clinical psychology, community paediatrics, school reports and the surgeon. Management options include non-surgical options (do nothing, taping the ears in young infants, psychotherapy, watch and wait) and surgical.

Be aware that surgery is increasingly subject to local funding restrictions and centralised to specialist centres. Ideal age for surgery is pre-school.

Tell me about the surgical options for this patient

> ☑ • Suture techniques e.g. Mustarde/Furnas
> • Cartilage scoring techniques e.g. Farrior/Chongchet
> • Combination techniques
> • Minimally invasive techniques e.g. Earfold device

Be able to describe a technique that you have seen or performed. Examiners are aware that you may not have performed this surgery, but you ought to still be able to describe a technique including incision site, suture choice and post-operative management.

What are the complications of pinnaplasty surgery?

- *Early*: Haematoma, bleeding, infection/perichondritis, skin necrosis, wound dehiscence
- *Late*: Scarring (including keloid/hypertrophy), suture extrusion, asymmetry between sides, hypoaesthesia, poor aesthetic result e.g. telephone ear, overcorrection of helix, narrowing of the EAC

Are you familiar with any non-surgical options for managing prominauris?

- Taping and moulding
- EarWell infant cradle: To hold the ear in the ideal position. The device is perforated to allow patients to hear
- EarBuddies: Splints used to remould the cartilage which are held in place with tape
- Earfold device: A nickel–titanium implant placed under LA

Septal Perforation

MARK FERGUSON

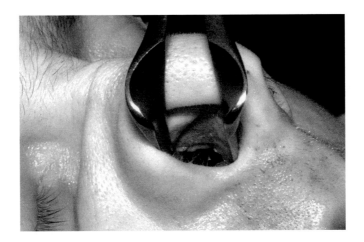

What does this photo show?

'This is a clinical photograph through the right nares showing a septal perforation'.

What is the likely underlying cause?

- Previous septal surgery
- Trauma
- Intranasal drug use
- GPA/vasculitis

There are many other possible causes, including malignancy, but these are the four most likely.

How do these patients present?

- Crusting
- Whistling
- Nasal obstruction
- Saddle nose deformity or nasal collapse
- Nasal/facial pain (cocaine/vasculitis can be painful)
- Referred by renal/rheumatology with known GPA

How would you investigate these patients?

In the history you would ask about:

 • Previous septal surgery
- Intra-nasal drug abuse. Note recent reports of cocaine induced vasculitis
- Pre-existing conditions e.g. GPA

In the examination you would look for:

 • Degree of tip support
- Nasal collapse
- Presence of saddle nose deformity

- Perform anterior rhinoscopy to visualise the location and size of the perforation as well as evaluating the condition of the nasal mucosa.
- Complement this with nasendoscopy to identify other concurrent pathology in nose e.g. polyps, and to look for laryngeal involvement of GPA.

 • Bloods: FBC, U&E, ESR, ANCA – PR3/MP0, ACE

- CT sinuses

If you are suspecting GPA, refer to renal physician as there is up to 30% mortality in the first year from untreated renal disease.

What are the treatment options?

If ongoing drug abuse – discuss behaviour change and consider involving drug and alcohol services.

Medical: Treat the underlying cause e.g. GPA (MDT with renal/rheumatology/ENT)

Nasal treatment:

- Antibiotic creams
- Normal saline douche

Surgical options

Say what your unit would do, for example:

Offer septal perforation repair endonasal/open +/− ear cartilage graft

Some units use septal buttons or silastic splints, which may be effective for some patients (approximately 40% success).

 Further reading:

Coordes A, Loose SM, Hofmann VM et al. Saddle nose deformity and septal perforation in granulomatosis with polyangiitis. *Clin Otolaryngol*. 2018 Feb;43(1):291–9. doi: 10.1111/coa.12977. Epub 2017 Sep 21.

Pereira C, Santamaría A, Langdon C et al. Nasoseptal perforation: From etiology to treatment. *Curr Allergy Asthma Rep*. 2018 Feb 5;18(1):5. doi: 10.1007/s11882-018-0754-1.

Septorhinoplasty

SAMIT UNADKAT

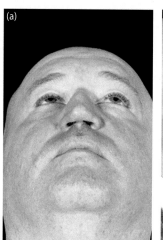 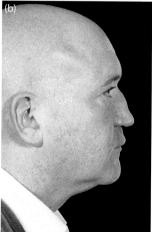

Please describe these photographs

'*The first is a clinical photograph of a middle-aged male patient in basal view demonstrating a widened nasal bridge, deviated nasal bony pyramid to the right and shortened columella. The second is a right lateral view demonstrating a pseudohump with a supratip saddle nose deformity. There is reduced columella show and mild ptosis of the tip. Ideally, I would like to examine the remainder of the photographs in line with the Institute of Medical Illustrators guidelines. As a minimum, I would like to see left and right lateral views, left and right oblique views, a frontal view, and a basal view*'.

Other views, including forced inspiration view, skyline view and smiling view can be taken, but avoid getting too fixated on every possible perspective.

The description ought to be a general overview and will be fairly obvious. It is not a comprehensive aesthetic assessment.

 Further reading:

- Nasolabial and nasofrontal angles and how they differ between men and women
- Frankfort plane (horizontal line from the cephalic tragus to the infraorbital rim in lateral view)
- Rule of horizontal thirds and vertical fifths in relation to the whole face

What would you like to ask in your history?

- What concerns the patient – function/aesthetics/combination
- Rhinorrhoea/post nasal drip
- Nasal blockage – unilateral, bilateral, alternating
- Bleeding/crusting/whistling
- Alteration in sense of smell – hyposmia, anosmia, parosmia, cacosmia
- Previous surgery or trauma
- Recreational drug use and smoking history
- Review of systems including respiratory, musculoskeletal or renal problems
- Occupation
- Body dysmorphia

How would you examine the nose?

- Inspection
  - Divide the nose into thirds (upper third: Nasal bones, mid third: Septum and ULC, lower third: Nasal tip and LLC)
  - Examine the nose in relation to the rest of the face (horizontal thirds and vertical fifths)
  - Look for obvious scars, skin changes or structural deformities. Comment on skin thickness
  - Resting inspiration to look for valve collapse
- Palpation
  - Tip recoil and irregularities of the nasal dorsum
- Anterior rhinoscopy
- Special tests
  - Modified Cottle's
  - Nasal inspiratory peak flow
  - Acoustic rhinomanometry
- Rigid nasal endoscopy

What are the causes of a supratip saddle nose deformity?

- Post-traumatic
- Infection e.g. previous abscess
- Previous surgery
- Vasculitis including sarcoidosis and GPA
- Post-radiotherapy
- Congenital

Be able to draw the nasal septum and mark the keystone area

Be aware that a saddle nose deformity may also have a concurrent septal perforation.

Given that this patient is complaining of left nasal blockage and has a deviated nasal septum and is also unhappy about the deviated bony pyramid, how would you surgically correct this deformity?

This will vary on your level of experience. Whilst it may be acceptable to say that you would refer this patient to a colleague, you ought to be able to describe the basic approach of either an open or an endonasal septorhinoplasty:

'Assuming that I have taken informed consent from the patient, I would like to undertake an endonasal septorhinoplasty through a left hemitransfixion incision and bilateral intercartilaginous incisions. After raising bilateral mucoperichondrial flaps, I would perform a septoplasty and harvest some cartilage for the augmentation. I would carry out medial and percutaneous lateral osteotomies and crushed cartilage onlay graft to augment the supratip area'.

Note, there are so many variations to answer this scenario and this is just one example. Stick to what you have done in your training and keep it simple. Make sure you listen carefully to the question being asked.

 Read about the incisions for an open vs. endonasal septorhinoplasty.

What are the risks of surgery?

 General

- Bleeding, infection, risks of anaesthesia

Specific

- Septal perforation/abscess/haematoma
- Numbness of the nasal tip and upper lip
- Bruising/crusting/swelling
- Failure to correct deformity
- Imperfect result/asymmetry
- Need for revision surgery (10%–15%)
- CSF leak
- Anosmia
- Scar – depending on the approach
- Adhesions

Be able to describe how you would manage a septal haematoma.

In the latter stages of the viva, if you are doing well, you may be asked more challenging questions:

- Major and minor tip support mechanisms
- Anderson's tripod theory
- Justifying open approach vs. endonasal approach to septorhinoplasty surgery

Sinonasal Tumours

MOHIEMEN ANWAR

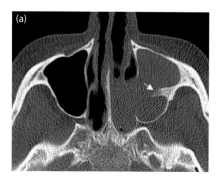 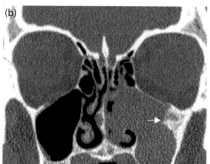

Describe these images

'The image on the left is a non-contrast axial CT scan on bone window through the level of the nose and maxillary sinuses, showing a completely opacified left maxillary sinus and soft tissue within the left nasal cavity. The arrow is pointing to a bony prominence within the left maxillary sinuses which might be just a normal structure or evidence of a new bone formation within the sinus. The image on the right is a non-contrast CT scan in the coronal plane and bone window at the level of the eye and sinonasal cavity. The left maxillary sinus is completely opacified with evidence of new bone formation and there is a soft tissue shadow within the left nasal cavity. The osteomeatal complex on the left is totally opacified. The mass is not causing any bony erosion, as evident by the intact lamina papyracea and intact skull base. Considering the finding of no bony invasion, but new bone formation, then this mass most probably represents a chronic process that is unlikely to be malignant, however I would like to exclude this by arranging an MRI of the sinuses and urgent EUA and biopsy of the lesion'.

In unilateral sinonasal disease, the discussion will start by reviewing an image of the scan. If the history is not provided, talk through the possible significant points e.g. unilateral nasal obstruction, unilateral epistaxis, sense of smell, smoking, occupation, weight loss and previous surgery. Offer examiners a differential diagnosis based on the scan analysis and history:

- CRS
- Antrochoanal polyp
- Benign sinonasal disease (e.g. inverted papilloma, mucocele)
- Malignant sinonasal disease

What is the advantage of MRI over CT in unilateral sinonasal pathology?

CT scan alone is not able to differentiate between a soft tissue mass and retained sinus secretions whilst MRI of the sinuses is able to delineate what is soft tissue mass and what is retained mucosal secretions. MRI of inverted papilloma reveals convoluted cerebriform-patterned mucosa.

Talk me through the management of antrochoanal polyp (ACP)

ACP is a single giant inflammatory polyp that arises from the mucosa of the maxillary sinus, most commonly arising from the postero-medial wall and extending through accessory ostia posteriorly into the post-nasal space.

The history is typically of a unilateral nasal obstruction in a young adult who is otherwise fit and well. Examination reveals a unilateral large nasal polyp on anterior rhinoscopy and nasal endoscopy. As the lesion is almost always unilateral imaging is indicated (CT sinuses).

Differential diagnosis:

- Inflammatory nasal polyposis
- Inverted papilloma
- Mucocele
- Sinonasal carcinoma

Treatment:

- Endoscopic sinus surgery with a large middle meatal antrostomy.
- In very rare circumstances a sub-labial Caldwell-Luc approach may be used for large ACP, although usually large polyps can be debrided first and removed endoscopically.
- Recurrence following complete resection is about 7%–10%.

It is worth being able to quote your unit's figures or a reference for this.

- In recurrence and revision cases, consider a large middle meatal antrostomy and stripping of maxillary sinus mucosa.

Prepare to discuss the disadvantages of this procedure in the shape of interfering with mucociliary clearance.

Be prepared to discuss some aetiological theories for the formation of ACP, the strongest evidence supports two theories:

- Underlying abnormality in the mucociliary clearance
- Difference in pressure across the maxillary antrum
- Idiopathic

There are other types of giant single polyp e.g. spheno-choanal polyp, the discussion should follow the same pattern as above.

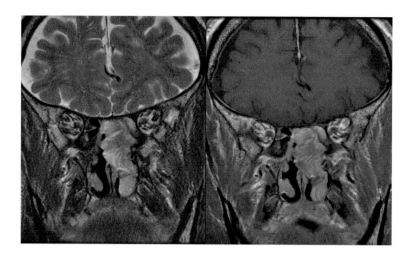

This is a further scan of the same patient. Please describe these images.

'These are images of a coronal MRI scan at the level of the sinonasal cavity. The image on the left is a T2 enhanced showing a mass arising from the left sinonasal cavity. The image on the right is a T1-enhanced image of the same patient. The lesion appears to be of soft tissue in nature and arising from the inferior turbinate. It has the typical cerebriform appearance on MRI that is highly suggestive of Schneiderian papilloma or inverted papilloma'.

Despite being benign, inverted papilloma has a high recurrence rate. Additionally, they carry a 5%–12% rate of transformation into SCC.

What is the mainstay of management of such tumours?

- Endoscopic excision, with or without medial maxillectomy (except for those that invaded frontal sinus, orbit or skull base) is recommended. It is most important that the resection is sub-periosteal and that all sclerotic bone is removed.

The European position paper on endoscopic management of tumours of the nose, paranasal sinuses and skull base recommends regular follow-up up to 3 years. It also recommends endoscopic management.

- The role of adjuvant radiotherapy is still unclear but discussion in an H&N or skull base MDT is important.

Are you aware of any grading system for inverted papilloma?

- Krouse classification
  - T1: Nose only
  - T2: Extend to ethmoid and maxillary
  - T3: Extend to frontal and sphenoid
  - T4: Bony destruction and beyond sinuses. Exclude malignancy

Skin Cancer

SAMIT UNADKAT

Please describe this photograph

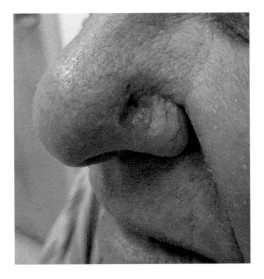

Image credit: Ananth Vijendren

'*This is a clinical photograph of a well circumscribed, pigmented lesion measuring approximately 1 cm over the left alar region of this patient's nose. The edges are rolled and pearly with evidence of surrounding telangiectasia in keeping with a likely BCC. My differentials would also include a melanoma and SCC*'.

What are the risk factors for developing skin cancer?

- Chronic sun exposure
- Fitzpatrick skin types I and II (fair skin)
- Other forms of ionising radiation
- Immunosuppression
- Previous skin malignancy
- Premalignant states e.g. multiple actinic keratoses

What are the different subtypes of BCC?

- Low risk: Nodular and superficial
- High risk: Morphoeic (infiltrative), micronodular and basosquamous

How would you manage this lesion?

'I am suspicious that this lesion is a BCC. After undertaking a full head and neck history and examination, I would ideally want to excise the lesion with a minimum of a 4–5 mm margin as it is a high-risk site. However, given its proximity to the alar margin, in this particular case, I would need a punch biopsy first as I am likely to need a local flap to close the resultant soft tissue defect. I am aware that dermoscopy also plays a role to aid the diagnosis though my experience is limited. Should the histological subtype be high risk, I would discuss this in my local skin cancer MDT and consider Mohs micrographic surgery. If it is low risk, I would proceed with a wide local excision with a 4–5 mm margin and reconstruct with a local flap such as a bilobed flap'.

> For high risk tumours, or greater than 2 cm, aim for a 13–15 mm margin if possible. For recurrent BCC, aim for 5–10 mm.
>
> Imaging for primary BCC is generally not required.

Can you tell me about the reconstructive ladder?

- Healing by secondary intention
- Direct or primary closure
- Delayed primary closure
- Skin grafts (split/full thickness)
- Tissue expansion
- Local flaps
- Distant flap
- Free flap

What is the blood supply of the bilobed flap that you are proposing?

It is a random transposition flap with no defined pedicle. The flap is supplied by musculocutaneous and cutaneous perforators.

What are the adverse prognostic features of a BCC?

- Size >2 cm
- Central face location
- Poorly defined margins
- High risk histological subtypes
- Perineural and perivascular involvement
- Immunosuppressed patient

What are the non-surgical options for BCC management?

 • Conservative – BCCs are often slow growing
- Curettage and cautery
- Cryosurgery
- Photodynamic therapy
- Topical 5% imiquimod
- Radiotherapy
- Vismodegib

If you are asked about recurrent or incompletely excised BCC, you are probably doing fairly well. Just remember to discuss these tricky cases in your skin MDT.

What is Mohs micrographic surgery?

'A surgical technique that excises a tumour sequentially at a 45-degree angle thereby providing total histological control of the surgical margins and maximal tissue preservation'.

What are the indications for Mohs micrographic surgery in the context of BCC?

- Infiltrative or morphoeic involving the face
- Invasive primary BCC (any subtype) where tissue preservation is desirable to facilitate reconstruction e.g. eyelids, vermilion border, alar margin
- Large >2 cm BCC of any subtype
- Invasive recurrent BCC

 Make sure you have read and know the latest UK guidelines on the management of BCC, SCC and malignant melanoma.

Index

Abbé flap, 266
ABI, *see* Auditory brainstem implants
ACC, *see* Adenoid cystic carcinoma
Accessory nerve, 45–46, 47
Achondroplasia, 226
Acoustic gain, 93
Acute myringotomy, 203
Acute sinonasal infections, 240–243
    examination, 241
    investigations, 241
    MDT for, 240
    orbital septum, 240
    patient history, 240–241
    Pott's puffy tumour, 242–243
    scan for, 241
    stage 5, in Chandler's classification, 242–243
    surgical intervention in, 241
Acute vestibular syndromes, 166
Adenoid cystic carcinoma (ACC), 75
Age-appropriate audiology, 211
Agger nasi cell, 257
AIED, *see* Autoimmune inner ear disease
Air conduction hearing devices, 92
    accessories, 93
    BTE, 92, 93
    extended wear hearing aid, 93
    types of, 92
Alar margin, full-thickness defect
    of, 263–264
Alexander's law, 163
Allergic fungal sinusitis, 271
Aminoglycosides, 124
Amphotericin, 272
Anaesthetics, 116
Anosmia
    causes of, 248–249
    examination, 248
    investigations, 248
    management, 249
    patient history, 248
Anti-fungals, 272
Anti-reflux therapy, 28
Apert syndrome, 225
Apnoea, 48
Arnold-Chiari malformation, 167
Aspergillus flavus, 127

Aspergillus fumigatus, 270
Audiograms, 132–133
Auditory brainstem implants (ABI), 100
Auditory rehabilitation options, 136
Autoimmune hearing loss, 150
    investigations for, 150–151
    treatment, 151
Autoimmune inner ear disease (AIED), 150

BAHA, *see* Bone anchored hearing aid
BAHI, *see* Bone anchored hearing implant/
    instrument
Battle's sign, 156
Belfast rule, 137
Bell's palsy, 118–120
Benign laryngeal lesions
    adjuvant medical treatments, 27
    aetiology, 27
    clinical findings, 26, 27
    malignant transformation, risk of, 26
    microlaryngoscopy, 28
    patient history, 26
    patient management, 26
    Reinke's oedema, 28
    vocal cord granuloma, 28
    vocal cord nodules, 28
    vocal cord polyps, 28
Benign paroxysmal positional vertigo
    (BPPV), 94
    causes of/risk factors for, 94
    CRM, 96
    diagnosis of, 95
    forms of, 94
    idiopathic, 95
    MRI for, 97
    natural patient history, 96
    patient history, 94
    posterior canal, 95
    post-manoeuvre recommendations, 97
    surgery, role of, 97
    tests for, 96
    theories, 94
Betahistine, 124
Betnesol-N, 116
BiCROS aids, 92
Bilobed flap, 266

Bluetooth devices, 93
Body worn aids, 92
Bone anchored hearing aid (BAHA), 98, 99
Bone anchored hearing implant/instrument
    (BAHI), 99
Bone conduction, 99
Bone conduction hearing devices, 98
    in children, age for, 100
    implant surgery, complications of, 99
    indications for, 99
    MEIs, 100
    osseointegrated fixtures in children with
        microtia, 100
    types of, 98
    in UK, 100
BPPV, *see* Benign paroxysmal positional vertigo
Brainstem ischaemia, 166–167
Branchial anomalies, 170
    branchial cleft anomalies, 171
    diagnosis of, 170
    embryological origin of, 170
    hearing loss, 171
    tonsil and, 171
    treatment, 170–171
Brandt-Daroff exercises, 95
BTE air conduction hearing aid, 92, 93

Caloric testing, 164
Canalithiasis, 94
Canalith repositioning manoeuvres
    (CRMs), 96
Canal-wall-down (CWD) approach, 107–108
Canal-wall-up (CWU) approach, 107–108
Candida species, 127
Canestan, 116
Carina, 101
Carotid body paragangliomas, 145
Cavernous sinus thrombosis, 242–243
Cerebellar testing, 20
Cerebellopontine angle tumours, 102
    diagnosis, 102–103
    management, principals of, 103–104
    vestibular schwanommas, 103
Cervical lymphadenopathy, 172
    differential diagnosis of, 173
    examination, 172
    open biopsy *versus* FNA-c, 173
    patient history, 172
    ultrasound for, 173
Chandler classification of periorbital cellulitis,
    218
CHARGE, 175
Chemotherapy, in head and neck cancer, 71

Choanal atresia, 174–177
    complications of surgery, 177
    embryology, 175
    initial management, 176
    investigations, 175–176
    nasal patency at bedside, assessment, 174–175
    patient history, 174
    stent insertion, 176–177
    surgical technique for treatment, 176
    syndromes associated with, 175
Cholesteatoma, 105
    acquired, 106
    canal-wall-up *versus* canal-wall-down
        approach, 107–108
    congenital, 105
    definition, 105–106
    endoscopic techniques for, 108
    extracranial, 106–107
    facial nerve monitoring for, 108–109
    intracranial, 106–107
    investigations, 107
    management of disease, 106
    mastoid obliteration techniques for, 108
    other considerations for, 109
    patient assessment, elements in, 106
    recidivism, monitoring for, 109
    untreated, complications of, 106
Cholesteatomas, 159
Chronic otitis media, 100–101
    assessment, 111
    CT scanning in, 111
    management options, 111
Chronic rhinosinusitis (CRS), 250
    in child, 251
    examination, 251
    patient history, 251
    surgery, benefits of, 252
    treatments, 252
    with/without polyps in adult, 250
Chronic vestibular syndromes, 166, 167
Chyle leaks, 67–68
CI, *see* Cochlear implants
Cleft lip and palate
    classification systems associated with, 178
    developmental abnormality for, 178
    diagnosis, 178
    ENT issues associated with, 180
    MDT cleft clinic, members in, 180
    risk factors, 180
    submucosal cleft, 181
    syndromes for, 179
    timeline for management, 180
CLOSET, 257

Clostridium difficile, 31
Cochlear implantation, 113
    factors for side of, 114
    function, 113–114
    interventions for, 114
    management, 114
    patient history for, 113
    process, 114–115
Cochlear implants (CI), 110
Congenital midline nasal masses, 182
    differential diagnosis, 182
    examination, 182–183
    investigations, 183
    management options, 183
    patient history, 182
Contact granuloma, *see* Vocal cord granuloma
Control of Noise at Work Regulations
        2005, 130–131
Co-phenylcaine, 116
Cranial nerve testing, 20
CRMs, *see* Canalith repositioning manoeuvres
CROS aids, 92
Crouzon syndrome, 225
CRS, *see* Chronic rhinosinusitis
CSF fistulae, 158
CSF rhinorrhoea, 253
    conservative management of, 255
    examination, 254
    imaging for, 254
    MRI signs of BIH, 254
    patient history, 253
    patient management, 254
    treatment of, 254
Cupulolithiasis, 94
Custom aids, 93

Deep neck space infections
    differential diagnosis, 29
    parapharyngeal abscess, 29, 29–30
        assessment of patient, 30
        differential diagnosis, 29, 30
        examination, 30–31
        investigation, 31
        patient history, 30
        patient management, 30–32
        treatment, 31–32
    risks associated with, 32
Depth of invasion (DOI), 53
Developmental milestones, 184–185
Dexamethasone, 154
Distortion, 93
Dix-Hallpike, 96
Dix-Hallpike positioning, 21

DOI, *see* Depth of invasion
Drooling, 186
    examination, 187
    investigations, 187
    management, 187
    patient history, 187
    salivary glands, 186
    severity, 186
    submandibular duct, relocation of, 187
    surgical options for, 187
DVAT, *see* Dynamic visual acuity test
Dynamic visual acuity test (DVAT), 164
Dysphagia, 66
    management, principles of, 66
    patient related outcome measures (PROMS) in, 66

Ear drops, 116
Electrocochleography (ECochG), 123
Electroneuronograph (ENoG) tests, 118
Endoscopic sinus surgery, 256–258
Endoscopic techniques, 108
*ENT OSCEs - A Guide to Passing the DO-HNS
        and MRCS (ENT) OSCE*, 11
Episodic vestibular syndromes, 166, 167
Epistaxis, 259–261
    management, 261
    patient history, 259–260
Epley manoeuvre, 95
Esthesioneuroblastoma, *see* Olfactory
        neuroblastoma
Ewald's law, 96
Extended neck dissection, 46
Extended wear hearing aid, 93
External ear canal stenosis, 159
Extracranial cholesteatoma, 106–107

Facial nerve, 117
    course of, 117
    monitoring, 108
Facial nerve injury, 158
Facial pain, 267
    characteristics of, 267
    differential diagnosis of, 267
    imaging for, 268
    midfacial segment pain, 268
    patient history, 267
    rhinosinusitis, symptoms of, 267
Facial palsy, 117–120
    causes of, 118–119
    grading classification systems of, 118
    prognosis of, 119
    surgical options for, 119–120
    treatment, 119

Fistula testing, 22
Forehead flap, paramedian, 263
FRCS (ORL-HNS) examination, 1–2
   four months pre-exam, 4
   one day pre-exam, 5
   one month pre-exam, 4
   one week pre-exam, 5
   part 1, general advice for preparing for, 3–6
   part 2, general advice for preparing for, 7
      cerebellar testing, 20
      clinical stations, 8–9, 11–24
      communication skills, 9
      cranial nerve testing, 20
      Dix-Hallpike positioning, 21
      ear examination, 11–13
      examination of balance, 15
      fistula testing, 22
      gait tests, 19–20
      hyperventilation, 22
      lateral brainstem dysfunction, tests of, 22
      oculomotor testing, 16–18
      oral cavity, neck, thyroid and parotid
         glands examination, 14–15
      oscillopsia testing, 22
      otoscopy and tuning fork tests, 22
      paediatric examination, 15
      rhinology and facial plastics examination,
         13–14
      vestibular testing, 18–19
      vivas, 7–8
   six months pre-exam, 3
   syllabus for, 1
   topics, 5–6
   two months pre-exam, 4
Frenzel glasses, 95
Fronto-ethmoidal cells, 257
Fungal sinusitis, 270
   classifications for, 270–271
   diagnostic criteria for, 271–272
   invasive, 270, 271
   mucormycosis, 271
   non-invasive, 270

Gait tests, 19–20
Gentisone HC, 116
Glomus tumours, *see* Paragangliomas
Goldenhar syndrome, 224
GOSH Paediatric Airway Sizing Chart, 209
Gray (Gy), 69

Haemotympanum, 156
Haller cell, 257

Halmagyi head-thrust test, 163
Hands-free headset, 93
Head shake test, 164
Health and Safety at Work Act 1974, 130
Hereditary haemorrhagic telangiectasias, 273
   blood vessels and, 275
   diagnostic criteria for, 273
   genetics, 275
   investigations, 274
   management, 274
   patient history, 273–274
Herpes zoster oticus, 166
HINTS acronym, 168
House-Brackmann 6-point scale, 118
HPV, *see* Human papillomavirus
Human papillomavirus (HPV), 27
Hyperventilation, 22
Hyperventilation test, 164
Hypocalcaemia
   post thyroidectomy
      investigations for, 34
      patient management, 34
   signs and symptoms, 34
Hypopharyngeal cancer, 35
   anatomical subsites of, 35
   patient history, 35
   patient management, 36
   PET-CT for, 36
   prognosis for, 37
   treatment options for, 36–37
Hypopnoea, 48

IAM, *see* Internal auditory meati
Idiopathic BPPV, 95
Infantile haemangioma, 235
Internal auditory meati (IAM), 123
International Society for the Study of Vascular
      Anomalies (ISSVA), 234
Intracranial cholesteatoma, 106
Invasive fungal sinusitis, 270, 271
Inverted papilloma, *see* Schneiderian papilloma
Isolated small incudostapedial erosion, 136
ISSVA, *see* International Society for the Study of
      Vascular Anomalies

JNA, *see* Juvenile nasopharyngeal angiofibroma
Jugulotympanic paraganglioma, 146
Juvenile nasopharyngeal angiofibroma (JNA),
      188
   differential diagnosis, 188–189
   Fisch staging system for, 189
   histology, 190–191

management, 189
patient history, 188
recurrence, 191
surgery for, 190

Karapandzic flap, 266
Keloids, 276
versus hypertrophic scar, 277
management of, 277
scar, 277–278
wound healing, stages of, 277
Kuhn cells, *see* Fronto-ethmoidal cells

Labyrinthine concussion, 166
Laryngeal cancer, 38
advanced, treatment options for, 41
investigation, 39
laser laryngeal surgery, classification system
for, 40
patient history, 38
treatment options, 39–40
T-staging of, 39
Laryngectomy stomal stenosis, 68
Laryngomalacia, 192
aetiology of, 193
anatomical features of, 193
coexisting comorbidities, 194
complications of, 193
investigations, 193
non-surgical treatment options for, 194
patient history, 192
severe, 192
supraglottoplasty
complications of, 194
steps of, 194
Lateral brainstem dysfunction, tests of, 22
Lignospan, 116
Lip flaps, 266
Locorten-Vioform, 116
Long process of incus (LPI), 110
LPI, *see* Long process of incus
Lund-McKay index score, 258
Lymphatic malformations, 236
Lymphoma, 173

Mal de debarquement (MdDS), 167
Masking
dilemma, 141–142
rules, 141–142
Mastoiditis, 203
Mastoid obliteration techniques, 108
MDADI, *see* MD anderson dysphagia inventory
MD anderson dysphagia inventory (MDADI), 66

MEIs, *see* Middle ear implants
Melkersson-Rosenthal syndrome, 119
Ménière's disease, 121, 166
classification, 122–123
diagnosis, criteria for, 122–123
differential diagnoses for, 122
and DVLA guidance, 125
investigations, 123
management, 123–125
patient history, 121–122
variants, 122
Methylprednisilone sodium succinate, 154
Microtia, 195
classification, 195
management, considerations in, 195–196
pinna reconstruction, 196
surgical hearing rehabilitation, 196
syndromes, 196
Middle ear implants (MEIs), 100
Möbius syndrome, 119
Modified radical neck dissection (MRND), 46
Moffatt's solution, 258
Mohs micrographic surgery, 297
MRND, *see* Modified radical neck dissection
Mucopolysaccharidoses, 225–226
Mucormycosis, 271
Multinodular goitre, 81
Myer-Cotton grading system for subglottic
stenosis, 207

Nasal dermoid, 182, 183
Nasal encephalocele, 182, 183
Nasal glioma, 182, 183
Nasal obstruction with dyspnoea in neonates,
174–177
Nasal tip, 262
reconstructive options for, 262–263
Nasolabial flap, 264
Nasopharyngeal cancer (NPC), 42
classification systems for, 43
clinical evaluation, 43
imaging investigations, 43
patient history, 42–43
staging, 43–44
surgery for treatment, 44
Neck dissections, 45–47
accessory nerve, 45–46, 47
classification, 46
complications of, 47
rationale for, 46
skeletonising and devascularising,
risk of, 47
skin incisions used for, 46

Neck trauma
    carotid artery injury, management of, 59–60
    classification, 58
    common vessels injured in, 59
    high-velocity injuries, 58
    immediate surgical management, indications
        for, 58
    low-velocity injuries, 58
    management, 59
    severe, management of, 58
    vascular injury, management of, 59
Necrotising otitis externa
    common pathogen in, 127
    definition, 126
    diagnosis of, 127
    imaging techniques for, 127
    patients management, 128
    presence, 127
Necrotising otitis externa (NOE), 119
Neonates, nasal obstruction with dyspnoea in,
        174–177
Nerve trauma, classification of, 117–118
NIHL, *see* Noise-induced hearing loss
NOE, *see* Necrotising otitis externa
Noise-induced hearing loss (NIHL), 129
    acute acoustic trauma, 130
    Control of Noise at Work Regulations 2005,
        130–131
    investigations for, 130
    management of, 130
    patient history, elements in, 130
Non-invasive fungal sinusitis, 270
Non-organic hearing loss, 132
    assessment, 134
    definition, 133
    management, 134
NPC, *see* Nasopharyngeal cancer
N2-3 SCC, 71

Obstructive sleep apnoea, 197
    adenotonsillectomy for, 198
    management, 197–198, 199
    patient history, 197
    sleep investigations, 198
Obstructive sleep apnoea (OSA)
    on driving, advise for patient, 49
    grade, 48
    management of, 49
    patient examination, 48
    patient history, 48
    sleep studies, 48–49
    surgical options for, 49
Occlusion effect, 93

Oculomotor testing, 16–18
Olfactory neuroblastoma, 279
    classification system for, 280
    differential diagnosis of, 280
    endoscopic surgery for, 281
    investigations of, 280
    management, 280
    patient history, 280
    patients followed-up, 281
    prognosis, 281
    surgery, contraindications for, 281
Onodi cell, 257
Oral cavity cancer, 50
    clinical assessment, 50
    ethnic origin, 50
    external beam radiotherapy for, 52
    mandibular cortex and, 51
    neck dissection for, 51
    past medical patient history, 50
    patients care, specialties for, 53
    pre-operative assessment, 50
    principles of reconstruction in oral surgery,
        52
    risk factors, 50
    staging, 50, 53
    treatment, 51
ORN, *see* Osteoradionecrosis
Oropharyngeal cancer, 54
    HPV-related, 55
    initial management, 55
    patient history, 54
    T2N2bM0 stage, 55
    TNM 8 staging, 56–57
OSA, *see* Obstructive sleep apnoea
Oscillopsia testing, 22
Osseointegration, 99
Ossiculoplasty, 135
    audiogram finding, 135–136
    auditory rehabilitation options, 136
    classification, 137
    complications of, 138
    footplate replacement, options for, 136
    ossicular reconstruction options, 136
    PORP *versus* TORP, 136, 137, 138
    as primary procedure, 136
Osteoradionecrosis (ORN), 52, 70
    mandibular, 70
Otic capsule disrupting, 157
Otic capsule sparing, 157
Otitis media, 201
    acute myringotomy, 203
    antibiotics for, 202
    assessment, 202–203

complications of, 202
mastoiditis, 203
patient history, 202
Otolithic function, 165
Otomize, 116
Otosclerosis, 139
differential diagnoses for, 140
dip in bone conduction, significance of, 139
investigations, 140
management, 140
masking dilemma and, 141–142
masking rules and, 141–142
patient history, 140
surgery, contraindications to, 141
Otoscopy and tuning fork tests, 22
Otosporin, 116
OVEMP, 165

Paediatric airway compromise, 204
adult *versus* paediatric airway, 206
adult *versus* paediatric tracheostomy, 207
biphasic stridor, 205–206
elevated respiratory rate, 205–206
examination, 204–205
Myer-Cotton grading system for subglottic
stenosis, 207
paediatric tracheostomy, decannulation
protocol for, 209–210
patient history, 204
stertor *versus* stridor, 205
Paediatric hearing loss, 211
assessment
objective tests, 214
subjective tests, 214–215
causes of, 212–213
and grommet insertion, 212
patient history, 212
and speech development, 212
test for, 211
type-B traces in both ears, 212
in UK, 213–214
Paediatric tracheostomy, decannulation protocol
for, 209–210
Paediatric tracheostomy tubes, 208
Paracusis of Willis, 140
Paragangliomas
aetiology, 145
assessment, 144
causes of, 145
classification systems for, 145–146
differentials, 143
examination, 144
hereditary, 145

jugular, 144, 145
management of, 146
patient history, 144
tympanic, 143, 144
types of, 144
vagal, 144
Paramedian forehead flap, 263
Parapharyngeal abscess, 29, 30
assessment of patient, 30
differential diagnosis, 29, 30
examination, 30–31
investigation, 31
patient history, 30
patient management, 30–32
treatment, 31–32
Parathyroid adenomas pre-op, 33–34
Pathophysiology, 70
Periorbital cellulitis, 216
Chandler classification of, 218
colour vision, assessment for, 217
common organisms for, 216
ENT UK guidance for medical treatment of,
217–218
imaging, indications for, 217
infection, spread of, 216
RAPD, assessment for, 217
sub-periosteal abscess, 219
Persistent postural-perceptual dizziness, 167
PET-CT scan, 82, 84
Pharyngeal pouch, 61
intervention, options for, 62–63
management, 62
patient history, 62
pouch size, classification system for, 63
surgery, complications of, 63
Pharyngocutaneous fistulas, 68
Pierre Robin sequence, 224
Pinnaplasty, 282
anatomical landmarks of, 283
complications of, 284
management options for, 283
non-surgical options for, 284
patient history, 283
surgical options for, 284
Plunging ranula, 72
PORT, *see* Post operative radiotherapy
Posterior canal BPPV, 95
Posterior diverticulum, 61
Post-laryngectomy care
dysphagia, 66
management, principles of, 66
patient related outcome measures (PROMS)
in, 66

Post-laryngectomy care (*Continued*)
  issues, 64
  speech types, 64
  surgical voice restoration
    primary, 66
    secondary, 66
    voice prostheses for, 66
  valve leakage problems, approach to, 65
Post-laryngectomy complications, 67
  chyle leaks, 67–68
  laryngectomy stomal stenosis, 68
  pharyngocutaneous fistulas, 68
Post operative radiotherapy (PORT), 52
Posturography, 165
Pott's puffy tumour, 243
Pre-auricular sinus, 147
  development of, 147
  differential diagnosis of, 148
  incidence, 148
  inheritance, 148
  recurrence, risk of, 148
  right ear, clinical photograph of, 147
  symptoms, 148
  treatment, 148
Presbyacusis, 149
  diagnosis of, 150
  hearing rehabilitation for, 150
  management options, 150
Primary hyperparathyroidism, 33
Proteus mirabilis, 127
P16 SCC, 84
Pseudomonas aeruginosa, 127
Pure tone audiogram, 149

Radical neck dissection (RND), 46
Radioactive iodine (RAI), 80
Radiotherapy, 69
  cells sensitivity to, 71
  Gray (Gy), 69
  indications for, 69
  side effects of, 70
  T3N0M0 larynx, regime in hospital for, 69
RAI, *see* Radioactive iodine
Ranulas, 72
  differential diagnosis, 73
  patient history, 72
  treatment options, 73
RAPD, *see* Relative afferent pupillary defect
Rapid Rhino nasal pack, 259
Recidivism, 109
Recurrent respiratory papillomatosis (RRP), 27, 220
  diagnosis, 220–221
  differential diagnosis, 220

multiple laryngeal papillomas, 220
  treatment options, 221
Reinke's oedema, 28
Relative afferent pupillary defect (RAPD), 217
Remote microphones, 93
Rhinitis
  intranasal medications for, 247
  management of, 244
  patient management, 246
  skin-prick allergy test for, 244–246
  steroid nasal sprays for, 247
  systemic steroids for treatment of, 246
Rhomboid flap, 264
RND, *see* Radical neck dissection
Romberg's test, 164
Rotational chair testing, 164
RRP, *see* Recurrent respiratory papillomatosis
Rules of masking, 141–142

Salivary gland malignancy, 74
  ACC, 75–76
  common neoplasms of, 76
  facial nerve, 76
  management, 75
  MRI, 75
  patient history, 74
  surgery, complications of, 75–76
Saturation sound pressure level, 93
Schneiderian papilloma, 294
Seddon's three-level classification
      system, 118
Selective neck dissection (SND), 46
Sensorineural hearing loss, 151
Sensory organisation test, 165
Septal perforation, 285
  causes, 285
  investigation, 286
  patient history, 286
  treatment options, 286
Septorhinoplasty, 288
  nose, examination of, 289
  patient history, 289
  risks of surgery, 290
  supratip saddle nose deformity, 289
Sialolithiasis, 77
  differential diagnosis, 77–78
  intraductal stone, management of, 78
  patient history, 77
  symptoms, 77
Sinonasal lamellae, 257
Sinonasal tumours, 292
  ACP, management of, 293–294
  MRI *versus* CT in, 293

Skin cancer, 295
    adverse prognostic features of, 296
    blood supply, 296
    management, 296
    Mohs micrographic surgery for, 297
    non-surgical options for, 297
    risk factors for, 295
    subtypes of BCC, 296
Skin graft, 264
Skin-prick allergy test, 244–246
Skull base, 258
SND, *see* Selective neck dissection
SNOT-22, 258
Sofradex, 116
SSCD, *see* Superior semicircular canal
      dehiscence
SSNHL, *see* Sudden sensorineural hearing loss
Staphylococcus aureus, 127, 242
Streaming accessories, 93
Sudden sensorineural hearing loss (SSNHL), 152
    definition, 152
    differential causes, 152
    examination for, 153
    follow up patient with, 155
    hearing rehabilitation, options for, 155
    intratympanic (IT) *versus* oral steroids,
      evidence for, 154
    investigations, 153
    management, 153–154
    oral steroids over placebo, evidence for, 154
    patient history, 153
    prognostic factors, 154
    treatment, 154
Sunderland's classification of nerve trauma, 117–118
Superior semicircular canal dehiscence (SSCD), 161
Supratip saddle nose deformity, 289

Temporal bone fracture, 156
    base of skull fracture, patient history for, 157
    cholesteatoma, 159
    classification of, 157
    with conductive hearing loss, 159
    external ear canal stenosis, 159
    management of patients with,157–159
    symptoms, 156
    with vascular injuries, 159
Thiazide diuretics, 123
Thy-grading, 80
Thyroglossal duct cyst, 227
    examination, 227
    patient history, 227
    surgical technique for, 228–229
    ultrasound for, 228

Thyroid cancer
    patient post-treatment for, 81
    RAI for, 80–81
Thyroid pathology, 79
    examination, 79–80
    follicular carcinoma, 80
    investigation, 80
    management, 80
    multinodular goitre, 81
    radioactive iodine (RAI), role of, 80
    symptoms, 79
    Thy-grading, 80
    thyroid cancer, patient post-treatment for, 81
    U-grading, 80
    U5 nodule, management of, 80–81
    vocal cord palsy, 80
Tinnitus, 160–161
Tonsillectomy
    assessment, 232–233
    complication of, 232
    indications for, 232
Tonsillitis, 230
    complications of, 231
    pathogens causes, 231
    treatment for, 231
Tonsils, 230
Treacher Collins syndrome, 224
Triadcortyl ointment, 116
Trisomy 21/Down syndrome, 222–224
T-tube, 111–112
Tympanometry, 203

U-grading, 80
Unknown primary cancer in head and neck,
      82–85
    benign squamous-lined cyst, 84
    differential diagnoses, 83
    immunohistochemistry tests, 84
    initial management, 82–83
    patient history, 83
    PET-CT in ENT, indications for, 83–84
    p16 positive SCC, 84
U5 nodule, management of, 80–81
Unterberger's/Fukuda's test, 164

Vascular anomalies, 234
Vascular injuries, 159
Vascular malformations, 234
    cutaneous, 235
    examination, 235
    infantile haemangioma, 235–236
    patient history, 235
    syndromes associated with, 237

Vascular tumours, 234
Velo-cardio-facial syndrome, 225
Vergence, tests of, 163
Vertigo, 162–168
    balance inputs, integration of, 163
    balance rehabilitation, role of, 165
    central *versus* peripheral cause, 168
    conditions, 165–168
    examination, 163
    eye movements assessment, 163–165
    nystagmus assessment, 163–165
    patient history, 162
    symptoms, 162
Vestibular migraine, 167
Vestibular neuronitis, 166
Vestibular schwanommas, 103
Vestibular testing, 18–19
Vestibulospinal reflex, 165
VHIT, 165

Vocal cord granuloma, 28
Vocal cord nodules, 28
Vocal cord palsy, 86
    bilateral palsy, 88–89
    causes of, 87
    injection materials, 88
    patient history, 86
    patient investigation, 87
    patient management, 87–88
    surgical options, 88
Vocal cord polyps, 28
V-Y advancement, 265

Wallerian degeneration, 118

Zenker's diverticulum, *see* Posterior
        diverticulum
Z-plasty, 265